the

wellness mama
5-step
lifestyle detox

the

wellness mama
5-step
lifestyle detox

THE ESSENTIAL DIY GUIDE TO A HEALTHIER,

CLEANER, ALL-NATURAL LIFE

Katie Wells

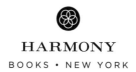

HARMONY

BOOKS · NEW YORK

Copyright © 2018 by Wellness Mama

All rights reserved.
Published in the United States by Harmony Books, an imprint of the Crown Publishing Group, a division of Penguin Random House LLC, New York.
crownpublishing.com

Harmony Books is a registered trademark, and the Circle colophon is a trademark of Penguin Random House LLC.

Wellness Mama and the Wellness Mama logo are trademarks/service marks of WellnessMama.com.

Library of Congress Cataloging-in-Publication Data has been applied for.

ISBN 978-0-451-49693-5
Ebook ISBN 978-0-451-49694-2

Printed in the United States of America

Book design by Elina D. Nudelman
Jacket design by Sarah Horgan
Jacket photographs: (bottle) M. PATTHAWEE/Shutterstock;
(lemon) Roman Somokhin/Shutterstock; (rosemary) domnitsky/Shutterstock

10 9 8 7 6 5 4 3 2 1

First Edition

TO TONY, IZZ, JOEY, GIGI, GABBI, GRETA, ALEXANDER, JEMMA, GEORGE, MARY CATHERINE, OLIVER, CASPIAN, WILLIAM, AND EVERY OTHER MEMBER OF THE NEXT GENERATION. MY HOPE IS THAT BOOKS LIKE THIS WILL HELP CHANGE THE WORLD FOR THE BETTER FOR YOU. YOU ARE THE HOPE FOR THE FUTURE.

CONTENTS

PART 3: *the recipes*

detox your life

As a mom to six kids and as a wife, my number-one priority is taking care of my family. I place a lot of importance on spending quality time with them and encouraging healthful lifestyles to keep us strong—emotionally and physically—and I want them to have everything they need to be safe, healthy, and happy.

But every time I turn around, the news is full of stories that scare me. One in five school-aged children (ages six to nineteen) has obesity, diabetes is on the rise in kids under age twenty, and toxins all around us can lead to autism, ADD, ADHD, asthma, cancer, and worse.

I remember reading an article ten years ago, after my first child was born, that this generation would be the first in centuries to have a shorter life expectancy than their parents. I was shocked by that statistic. I wanted better for my children and future generations!

A CRAZY, TOXIC WORLD!

It's sometimes confusing to know what to do. For one thing, there's all this crazy, conflicting advice about food. Not a week goes by without some miracle food or supplement being touted as the cure for everything from acne to cancer. The companies shilling these products have all kinds of flimsy studies to back up their claims and testimonials from people who insist they are cured.

At the same time, we continue to be sold fake food filled with chemicals, which takes the place of real food. The list of ingredients on many food labels often reads like something you'd see on a paint can.

The beauty and health industry is the same. The products are so chemical laden that I wonder if these are skin creams or something to kill bugs with. What are we exposing our bodies to day after day? The chemicals in our household products just add to the overload. And each time we step out the door we are exposing our bodies to environmental toxins and pollution.

Stress is toxic too. Life today sometimes seems like we're on a runaway train. Our busy, techno-driven culture takes a lot of our attention. We're glued to our smartphones, laptops, computers, and tablets, fulfilling our perpetual need to keep up with the constant flow of information while ignoring our already dwindling family life.

It's no wonder we struggle to adequately do the most important yet most difficult job we have: directing, managing, and being responsible for the outcome of our family.

PARENTS HAVE THE POWER TO CHANGE THE WORLD

That's too bad, because we, as parents, have tremendous power. We often forget it among the dirty dishes and the sleepless nights, but we are perhaps the strongest potential force for good in this world.

Day in and day out, we are raising the next generation. The world changers. The thought leaders of tomorrow. The people who will hopefully fix all the problems that past generations have caused. It is both a tremendous responsibility and an incredible gift.

We also control the majority of the purchasing power in our country and have the ability to shift the supply and demand of the food supply. When we vote with our dollars and our time, big companies take notice and make changes.

Look at the past decade's billion-dollar markets in natural products. We're demand-

ing healthier options for our families, and some companies are listening. At the same time, we're racing the clock on fixing health problems and environmental problems that threaten to change life as we know it.

MY STORY, MY PASSION

This is serious business, and it can create a lot of anxiety and illness. I know because I used to have serious health problems. I felt sick and draggy all the time, raising my many small children and dealing with a whole lot of stress. It took seven years and eight doctors to figure out what was wrong with me: Hashimoto's thyroiditis—an autoimmune disease that affects my thyroid. I knew I had to make changes, but there were so many conflicting opinions on how to go about it. It took me a long time to fully recover, but thanks to living more naturally, I am no longer sick. I know all too well what autoimmune disease feels like, and I don't want it for my children or for any other child.

Looking back, though, I'm forever grateful for this health struggle. Without it, I would never have learned about natural living or how to raise my children to have a healthier future.

You see, I'm a Type A, solution-side person who takes things in her own hands, goes on the offensive, and gets control over the seemingly uncontrollable. And so I became a mom on a mission: to make sure my family stayed healthy and happy—and with as little exposure to toxins and chemicals as possible—through natural living.

There was a lot of trial and error involved in creating a healthful natural lifestyle for my family. But finally, with my increasing concern about the toxicity of modern life, I was reborn as the Wellness Mama—a blogger, author, mom, and wife—determined to make natural living and real food doable, even with a big family and lots of distractions.

For starters, I committed to serving real food to my family—food that comes out of the ground and not out of some enticing box or package. I also decided to switch from using commercial household and personal products to ones I made myself. There are far too many chemicals in commercial products; they just weren't for me. Using basic, everyday ingredients, you can make effective, nontoxic cleaning products whenever you need them. All you need are a few simple on-hand items, such as baking soda, vinegar, lemon, and soap. This helps save money, time, and unnecessary packaging and offers a nice alternative to the harsh chemicals many cleaning products include.

Then I took on cosmetics. Like every other woman, I loved cosmetics, and I liked to slather creams on my face and body Eventually, I wised up to all the potentially toxic chemicals in this stuff. So I tried making my own cosmetics. The more I experimented, the more I became convinced that the most nourishing things you can put on your skin can be the same as those you put in your mouth. I started off using fruit—bananas, strawberries, whatever I had. I'd just get the blender out, throw them in, and rub them on. Soon, my skin and body were feeling and looking healthier than ever. My hair shined again. My face got radiant. Best of all, this cost almost nothing.

I also started making my own medicinal remedies to treat everything from colds to eczema to hair loss. If you came into my kitchen, for example, you might find me dabbing my finger in a mixing bowl filled with what looks like thick frosting. I'm not whipping up a dessert but rather a eucalyptus oil mixture to put on my daughter's chest to break up congestion.

I detoxed my life and my family's life from everything in the environment—including food—that might be harming us.

I decided that I didn't really want to go back to anything chemical based.

FIVE STEPS FOR DETOXING YOUR LIFE

Which brings me to this book: *The Wellness Mama 5-Step Lifestyle Detox*. It codifies everything I do in my life and work. It lays out step-by-step everything I'd do again in the quest for a more natural life with less exposure to chemicals in our environment. I also share some ways I went wrong in the hopes that you can learn from my mistakes and save time. My hope is that the detox will help you live a more natural, healthful life.

There are five steps in all; they help you flush toxins from your diet, create healing remedies in your own kitchen, make natural cosmetics and toiletries, banish harsh chemicals from your home, and free yourself from toxic stress—with other pieces of natural living advice peppered throughout.

Detoxing your entire life can sound intimidating, but if you take it gradually, step-by-step, you can do it. Try to stick to the plan; I've been doing it for so long now that natural living is second nature. The ultimate goal of the five-step program is to empower you to take control and enact change for your family, wherever it's needed the most. You don't have to do all five steps at once either. Simply start with the step you feel will make the most impact on your life, and then follow up with another step, then another, and pretty soon you'll be living naturally for the rest of your life, and so will your family. There are mini-steps grouped under each of the major steps, making it simple to point yourself in the right direction. Here's an overview:

Step 1, Give Your Body a New Start, is about detoxing your nutrition. This is not a diet but a look at what we all should be eating (or not eating) for lifelong health. You'll also learn how to do some simple meal planning, whether your family is small or large like mine. Food is always the best medicine, and in this step I show you how to turn food and herbs into truly curative remedies that will save you trips to the pharmacy. A study commissioned by the maker of a children's over-the-counter all-natural kids' respiratory and sinus medication concluded that an increasing number of moms are seeking out natural remedies to keep their children healthy. The poll found that 46 percent of the parents surveyed expressed an interest in natural remedies for their children.

Step 2, Enhance Your Beauty Regimen, is the logical progression from thinking about what you put *in* your body to thinking about what you put *on* it. We'll talk about how to look your best with natural cosmetics you can whip up in your kitchen. With so many chemicals in our toiletries and makeup, the alternatives included in this step are so important to total body health. Not only will you "save face," skin, and hair, you'll save money too.

Expect to be surprised by how little time it takes to make your own cosmetics. Forget bathroom cabinets full of expensive lotions and potions. In fact, everything you need to keep you looking young and beautiful can be found in your kitchen. Cooking oil can become part of your body lotions. Fruit is turned into cleansers and masks. Sugar and honey make terrific exfoliants and draw toxins from your skin.

In Step 3, Clean Up Without Chemicals, I introduce you to ways in which you can detox your home. After all, it should be your haven, a place where you should feel safe and relaxed, not harried and stressed out. I've got simple tips up my sleeves to help you get rid of chemicals, freshen the air, and restore restful energy to every room in your house.

Step 4, Do a Digital Detox, is about taking a technological fast—cutting back on time spent on smartphones, computers, tablets, and social media. Don't worry; you don't have to start the good-bye process cold turkey. I've got some surprisingly easy ways you can pull this off, which will let you spend more time with your family and enrich your family life exponentially.

Finally, in Step 5, De-stress to Detox, we look at the *s*-word—*stress*—with simple recommendations for dealing with it, from enjoying the outdoors to easy ways to fit exercise into your family's lifestyle. Additionally, you'll learn how restoring restful nights to your life helps your body naturally resist stress.

I wrap everything up with my life detox recipes—every formula, remedy, and concoction you need to make natural living your way of life. The power of these recipes is that they are toxin-free, and they work.

The tide is turning toward a more natural way of living, and DIY can be fun. If you can make a body lotion with a couple of ingredients, not only will it cost less, you'll know exactly what's going into it.

By the time we're done—and you have incorporated even just a few of these alternatives into your life—you'll know how to detox and live naturally.

Serve the best "clean" foods to your family and get your family to love those foods—making everyone feel fantastic. This is important! Studies show that when kids switch from sugary, additive-laden diets to fresh foods and natural alternatives, behavior improves, concentration increases, and immunity against common childhood illnesses is strengthened.

Make medicines with food and herbs. If anyone does get sick in your family, you'll have a whole natural medicine cabinet full of ways to banish things like sniffles, coughs, colds, and other nagging but common ailments that strike.

Keep your face, hair, body, teeth, and gums healthy the natural way. I want to know exactly what I'm rubbing on my skin, just as I want to know what I'm putting in my mouth—which is why I encourage people to make their own cosmetics. This can be super easy. If you can make a salad dressing or melt chocolate, you can make your own cosmetics.

Clean your house and purify your air without dangerous chemicals. You'll cut down on the amount of pesticides, allergens, and contaminants (not to mention grime) in your home by making your own natural cleaning products. I'll also arm you with invaluable knowledge about how to have the purest, healthiest drinking water in your home—since water is one of our most essential nutrients.

Go on a digital fast. Technology is wonderful, but as with anything, too much is not a good thing. Overdosing on digital devices and social media has been scientifically shown to hurt attention span and memory, disrupt family communication, and isolate people from real connections. You'll come to appreciate how a little distance between you and technology can create newfound serenity.

De-stress in a stressful world. This is really as simple as getting outdoors more often, doing simple exercises, and creating a better sleep environment, so that you literally resist stress. Take even a few of these actions, and you'll experience peace of mind, joy, and a confident attitude to carry you through life.

CREATING A BETTER WORLD FOR OUR CHILDREN

As a parent, you are the pillar of your household. You hold everything together, and you hold it high. So the more you can do for your own health, the better everyone else will feel.

As my friend Naveen Jain is fond of saying, we should strive not just to leave the world a better place for our children but to leave our children better for the world.

We're nearing the point of no return, but you and I have the power to pull our world back from the brink of these massive problems. Little changes you make for the better with your own family create ripples that can have a massive impact. Together, we really do have the power to change the world—and we must.

Solidly commit to trying a few of the basics here, then try even more—and you'll really change your life. The tools in this book, everything you need to raise your family well, and in wellness, will allow you to give your family the greatest gift—the gift of health.

Katie Wells, Wellness Mama

the preparation

what we're up against

I've always considered our bodies like a bathtub. You can put a lot of stuff into a bathtub. You can just add water, which is nonthreatening and easy to drain. You could add sand, or dirt, or fruit, or chemicals, or rocks, or any other substance really. No matter what you put in it, it has a maximum capacity.

Once that bathtub is filled to the top, it is going to overflow, no matter what you put into it. It is the same with our bodies. You can put a whole lot of different stuff into (and on) it and our bodies are pretty good at draining and cleaning out the junk. But if it's full of toxins, then the body can no longer drain it out and disease will manifest.

Our bodies can handle only so much. In their day, our grandparents weren't trying to put too much into the bathtub. Their bodies could relatively easily drain and stay below capacity, even if there was a large influx in a short amount of time.

Now we're throwing junk into the bathtub all day long. We're cramming it with plastics and chemicals and junk food and slowing down the drain with lack of sleep, too much stress, and lack of real human connection.

To fix it, we must reduce all the junk we're throwing in and address the draining issues. But before I get into that, let's delve into what we're up against (what's going into our bathtubs) so that you can understand how to combat it.

FOOD ADDITIVES

There are thousands of chemicals in our foods, and some experts estimate that consumers eat about four pounds of chemicals annually.

Sure, some additives are harmless, but others haven't been adequately tested and a bunch are downright dangerous. After looking into this issue, I've compiled a list of the ten most dangerous.

1. **Artificial Sweeteners.** Anything dubbed "sugar-free" probably contains artificial sweeteners, none of which have any redeeming value. I'm talking about aspartame, saccharin, acesulfame potassium, and others. These have been linked to cancer and a number of other serious health problems.

2. **Cochineal Extract.** Found in beverages, candy, ice cream, and yogurt, this additive is a red coloring made from the dried and pulverized bodies of insects. It has been shown to cause rare allergic reactions that range from hives to life-threatening anaphylactic shock.

3. **High-Fructose Corn Syrup (HFCS).** Found in almost all processed foods and beverages, this highly refined form of sugar is the chief source of calories in American diets. HFCS promotes obesity faster than many other sugars, builds up levels of low-density lipoprotein—LDL ("bad") cholesterol—and promotes the development of type 2 diabetes and other illnesses.

4. **Monosodium Glutamate (MSG).** A flavor enhancer found in soups, salad dressings, snack foods, chips, frozen meals, and many restaurant dishes, MSG is an "excitotoxin," meaning that it overstimulates brain cells to the point of damage or cell death. Studies show that regularly consuming MSG triggers depression, mental disorientation, fatigue, headaches, obesity, and other adverse side effects.

5. **Partially Hydrogenated Oil.** This is a type of vegetable oil hardened into a semisolid (such as shortening or margarine) by chemically adding hydrogen. This process creates trans fats, which can damage cell membranes. They also raise LDL cholesterol levels and lower high-density lipoprotein—HDL ("good") cholesterol—levels. This additive is found in many food products, including baked foods, microwave popcorn, piecrust, shortening, and stick margarine.

6. **Food Dyes.** These artificial colorings are used in soda, fruit juices, salad dressings, and other foods and have been linked to behavioral problems in children. According to a study funded by the British government and published in 2003, coloring agents in foods can cause kids to become hyperactive and disruptive. The UK Asthma and Allergy Research Center looked into the impact of artificial colorings on 277 three-year-olds over a two-week period. Researchers monitored the kids' behavior over the next two weeks, during which time the children were given placebos. Parents were asked to fill out assessment forms to track any significant differences in the children's behavior. Guess what? Parents observed substantial improvements when their children were not ingesting artificial colors. The researchers concluded that "significant changes in children's hyperactive behavior could be produced by removing colorings and additives from their diet."

7. **Sulfites.** These are preservatives used to increase shelf life in processed foods. According to the US Federal Drug Administration (FDA), approximately one in one hundred peo-

ple is sensitive to sulfites in food. Side effects include headaches, respiratory problems, and skin irrigations. In severe cases, sulfites can actually cause death by shutting off the airway altogether, leading to cardiac arrest.

8. **Sodium Nitrate and Sodium Nitrite.** Used as preservatives as well as for coloring and flavor in bacon, hot dogs, lunch meats, corned beef, and other processed meats, these substances can turn cancer causing once they enter the digestive system.

9. **BHA (butylated hydroxyanisole) and BHT (butylated hydroxytoluene).** Both preservatives are found in cereals, chewing gum, potato chips, and vegetable oils. They have been found to harm the neurological system of the brain, alter behavior, and increase the risk of cancer.

10. **Potassium Bromate.** This is a "dough conditioner" that plumps up volume in breads and rolls. It has been found to cause cancer in animals. Even small amounts can be harmful for humans.

wellness mama detox solution: Reduce or completely cut out the processed foods you normally purchase. Switch to a nutrition plan that consists of natural, organic foods, and always read labels. The more chemical ingredients in a food product, the less healthful it is. I feel happy when I feed my family quality food that avoids unnecessary harmful food additives—and so will you. Want to learn more? Visit WellnessMama.com and click on Health to read more about food and health topics.

PESTICIDES AND HERBICIDES

Each day, we encounter countless pesticides and herbicides, especially on food and even in our home environment. Of course, many are on our fruits and vegetables (unless you buy organic produce). There are too many to mention here, but there are two you should know about: 2,4-D and glyphosate.

The most commonly used weed killer for lawns and gardens, 2,4-D has been linked to cancer, neurological impairment, and reproductive problems. It is an "endocrine disruptor," a substance that wreaks havoc on weight, metabolism, and even fertility. Incidentally, 2,4-D was also a poisonous constituent of Agent Orange, which was used by the United States in the Vietnam War to defoliate jungles to expose hidden enemy installations.

It turns up in those weed-and-feed products you've probably bought hundreds of times to treat your lawn. Also problematic: 2,4-D lingers in the environment. It can drift by wind from the fields where it is sprayed to other places or be tracked inside homes by pets or kids. An analysis by the US Environmental Protection Agency (EPA) found 2,4-D in groundwater and surface water, as well as in drinking water.

wellness mama detox solution: This chemical has not yet been banned; until that happens, I suggest contacting a lawn service company that uses natural methods to control weeds on your lawn. Other good moves:

Avoid gardening and lawn care products that contain it.

Ask your municipality whether 2,4-D is used in local parks or outdoor recreational areas.

Check out the website of the National Pesticide Information Center, which has information on 2,4-D and most other pesticides. If you think anyone in your household has been exposed to 2,4-D or any other pesticide, contact a poison-control center.

Another scary chemical is glyphosate, the world's best-selling weed killer. Developed and patented by Monsanto, it is the active ingredient in the company's flagship herbicide Roundup. This product is a weed killer that consumers can use on their lawns. It is also sprayed on genetically modified crops, including soy, corn, cotton, canola, and sugar beets.

The authors of an MIT report have expressed concern that Roundup is contributing to a wide range of diseases, including inflammatory bowel disease, cancer, infertility, cystic fibrosis, cancer, Alzheimer's disease, and Parkinson's disease. The report notes that it "may be the most biologically disruptive chemical in our environment."

wellness mama detox solution: Eating organically grown foods and non–genetically modified foods is one important way to avoid the cocktail of synthetic chemical pesticides and excessively large amounts of glyphosate. Another is to grow your own veggies (see Chapter 5).

COSMETIC CHEMICALS

The twenty-first-century woman unknowingly applies hundreds of chemicals to her body every day. And the skin, as the body's largest organ, absorbs about 70 percent of whatever it comes into contact with.

Cosmetics and beauty products are thus a major source of chemical exposure for most people. An average beauty product contains dozens of harmful chemicals, many of which have not even been tested for safety in humans. So, what should you avoid?

- **Synthetic Fragrances.** Although they may make products smell good, they often contain phthalates, harmful chemicals added to stabilize and preserve fragrance oils and make plastic more durable. Phthalates mimic hormones and may alter genital development, particularily in boys.

- **Parabens.** Found routinely in skin care products, parabens act as preservatives and extend a product's shelf life. They also have hormone-altering side effects. Fortunately, many companies are eliminating them from their products.

- **Dioxane.** This is a chemical carcinogen used as a solvent in the production of many products. Exposure can cause damage to the liver, kidneys, and nervous system. To avoid it, watch out for any product containing these additives: myreth, oleth, laureth, ceteareth, polyethylene, polyethylene glycol, polyoxyethylene, or oxynol.

- **Sulfates.** These are usually labeled as sodium lauryl or sodium laureth. Both are harsh detergents put into products such as cleansers, soaps, and shampoos in order to create lather. Sulfates are derived from petroleum or vegetable oils that can be contaminated with pesticides. Sulfates can irritate eyes and cause skin rashes.

- **Petrochemicals.** They are derived from crude oil, the same stuff your gasoline comes from.

- **Artificial Colors.** You hear more about these as additives to food, but they're also in beauty products and thus can be absorbed by the skin. Clinical studies have found that most of them can cause cancer in animals.

- **Products Requiring Animal Testing.** A long and sad history of cruelty to animals lies behind many cosmetics. Look at it this way: If it had to be tested on animals in the first place, it probably isn't good for your skin.

wellness mama detox solution: The very best alternative is to make your own beauty and self-care products. In Step 2, I share the basic principles of creating a natural beauty routine from head to toe. Check out my natural beauty recipes in Chapter 19. You can also check out my full guide of safe beauty products and snag the ingredients to make your own at Wellness Mama.com/detox-book/.

ANTIBACTERIAL AGENTS

Antibacterial soaps and lotions are popular, feeding into our obsession with being germ-free. But there are serious problems with these products. Researchers now suspect that they may be involved in creating antibiotic-resistant superbacteria that have the potential to harm the population on a larger scale, and one way is by causing a buildup of dangerous staph bacteria in the nose and other parts of the body. This increases the risk of infection, amputation, and even death (especially after surgery).

If you have thyroid problems or other types of hormone imbalances, like I had, it turns out that antibacterial chemicals could be one contributing factor. Several studies have revealed that triclosan (the active ingredient in these products) can disrupt the body's ability to uptake thyroid hormone and can interfere with other hormone processes in the body. This hormone imbalance can lead to more advanced problems like infertility, obesity, and several cancers.

Widespread use of antibacterial chemicals, especially in hand soaps, has led to these chemicals getting washed down drains and into the water system. Studies show that these chemicals can remain, even after water treatment, and these chemicals (and many others, including plastic-based chemicals) are still found in streams and waterways around the world.

wellness mama detox solution: The good news is that regular soap and thorough hand washing works just as well as antibacterial products to get rid of germs. I've found that the best and least expensive way to avoid antibacterial chemicals is to make my own soaps and hand-washing sprays from coconut oil (which is a natural antiviral) and olive oil. Overall, just avoid any product touted as antibacterial, antiseptic, or antimicrobial and check out the list of safe soaps at WellnessMama.com /detox-book/.

INDOOR POLLUTANTS

It's sad to realize that indoor air can be more toxic than outdoor air—and often is! When analyzed, most household air tests positive for more contaminants than outdoor air. This is partially because of all of the chemicals in beauty products, household cleaners, air fresheners, and even furniture.

You may be shocked to learn that among

the worst indoor polluters are the scented candles you've probably lit hundreds of times. They give off chemicals considered as dangerous as secondhand smoke (another terrible health-damaging polluter). One of the chief offending substances in candles is paraffin wax. When burned, it creates highly toxic benzene and toluene—two known carcinogens.

What's more, many scented candles also have wicks that contain toxic metals such as lead. Even a few hours of burning them can release lead and other heavy metals into the air at levels that are much higher than acceptable limits.

wellness mama detox solution: Thankfully, we candle lovers have a great alternative: beeswax candles, which are not only safe but have the added benefit of helping clean indoor air.

VOLATILE ORGANIC COMPOUNDS

Volatile organic compounds, or VOCs, are chemicals that form a gas or vapor (fumes) at room temperature; they are given off by certain types of paints, scented candles, laundry detergents, and air fresheners.

VOCs are particularly harmful for babies and toddlers and can cause nausea, asthma, and damage to the nervous system.

wellness mama detox solution: Avoiding products that emit VOCs is the best move you can make. At the least, use paints that expressly say they are low VOC. Use essential oils (see pages 20–21) rather than air fresheners, and learn how to make your own laundry detergents. You can find recipes in Chapter 19.

HOUSEHOLD CLEANING PRODUCTS

Potential health threats lurk in the products we use around the house, most of which are laced with harmful, unapproved, and untested chemicals. In fact, the average household product contains more than sixty chemicals!

There is no federal regulation of household products, and manufacturers don't even have to disclose all of the ingredients in these products or list which ones are harmful! They don't have to provide safety data, nor do they have to perform any safety testing prior to marketing and selling these products.

Two of the worst cleaning products are chlorine and ammonia. You might have chlorine in your laundry room right now. But it's in other places too: drugs, computer chips, dry-cleaning compounds, laundry bleach, swimming pools, and drinking water. Why is it bad? Some recent studies show that chlorine can either mimic or block the body's natural hormones, especially the female hormone estrogen.

Ammonia is a very harsh chemical used in many household cleaners, including drain cleaners, oven cleaners, and toilet bowl cleaners. Contact with these chemicals can burn the eyes and skin and damage the throat and esophagus if accidentally swallowed.

wellness mama detox solution: Step 3 provides cleaning alternatives to chlorine and ammonia. Once you start making your own cleaning supplies with simple substances like white vinegar and baking soda, your home will gradually become chemical-free. Find my easy reference list of ingredients and safe cleaners at WellnessMama.com/detox-book/.

PLASTICS

Plastic products contain additives to make them more durable or pliable. One of the worst is BPA (bisphenol A), known to disrupt hormones and mimic the effect of estrogen in the body, leading to weight gain and hormone imbalances. It is widely known that plastics from food packaging can leach into food, which enters the body when consumed. The Centers for Disease Control and Prevention (CDC) reported that more than 92 percent of people who were tested, including newborn babies, had detectable levels of BPA and other plastic chemicals in their bodies.

Another scary ingredient found in plastics (and indoor air) are phthalates. These substances are considered to be especially harmful to men and boys, especially those who've been exposed to them in the womb. They are linked to immune system impairment, reduced testosterone, male infertility, and many other problems.

wellness mama detox solution: It's important to reduce our exposure to chemicals in plastics. Some recommendations:

Use glass or stainless-steel water bottles in place of disposable plastic water bottles (this is my favorite). Even better, fill your water bottle from a reusable stainless-steel water filter that will also help reduce chemical exposure from water.

Switch to reusable grocery bags instead of plastic or paper bags. These are widely available at many stores or you can make your own from old T-shirts. Bring lightweight mesh bags to the store to use for produce.

Stop buying processed foods that are packaged in plastics. This is a huge step for your health on its own, but it will also reduce the amount of plastic waste we produce each year. Shop at farmers' markets and bring reusable bags. If it is in a plastic bag or a box, just don't buy it.

LIFE TOXINS

If only those were all the problems! On top of the problems with our food supply and the chemicals in our environment, there are "life toxins" that also work against us as we try to be healthy. These invisible forces add to our "bathtubs" and increase the problems we face. These include:

Digital Overload. There are toxic problems emerging from our technological culture. Blue light, emitted from smartphones and computers, wrecks your sleep. Radio frequency waves from smartphones may cause cancer. And hovering over a smartphone or tablet all day can darken your mood.

Social Media. Kids, teens, and adults spend more time than ever online. When too many relationships are managed virtually, we miss out on the nuances of communication and emotional understanding that happen in live relationships.

Inactive Lifestyles. Kids and families today are getting a lot less exercise than the generations before us. One reason has to do with children spending so much time in front of a TV or computer screen. This means that kids burn fewer calories than if they were out playing sports or having outdoor fun. And sometimes all of us are just lazy or feel too busy to get some physical activity.

Health professionals are well aware that obesity—which can be caused by inactivity—increases the risk for a range of chronic diseases in adults. But the health of children can be hurt by their weight too. As I mentioned earlier, experts are claiming that childhood obesity leads to type 2 diabetes and even heart disease—which is why parents might outlive their kids in the future.

Lack of Sleep. Between 25 percent and 30 percent of normal kids and teens and adolescents are not getting enough sleep consistently, estimates the National Sleep Foundation. This causes poor attention, bad grades, school absences, poor social interactions, irritability, depression, increased automobile accidents, and more risk-taking behaviors. As for adults, poor-quality sleep is linked to stroke, Alzheimer's disease, heart problems, and obesity.

wellness mama detox solution: Don't feel overwhelmed. I've devoted two steps in this book to help you detox from these life pressures and situations. Every one of these life toxins can be tackled with a few easy-to-implement natural living strategies.

At this point, you might be mentally defaulting to the "Oh, please, everything is going to kill us . . . this is so alarmist and fear inducing"

mind-set, and I don't blame you. It is hard not to feel like everything is out to get us sometimes, but I truly believe many of these toxic exposures might be the "cigarettes" of our generation.

It was once considered absurd that smoking could be bad for you; there were even campaigns claiming that more doctors preferred one brand of cigarettes to another. And once upon a time, regulatory agencies declared now-banned chemicals like DDT safe for use. There were even ad campaigns promoting their usage around kids. So basically, a lot of stuff considered "okay" or even healthful way back when is now considered harmful, even lethal. Perhaps that is how we will think of these toxins in just a couple of decades. I hope so!

The good news is that little changes, like those you'll learn about in this book, can make a big difference over time. Take baby steps toward change when you have the time. Or experiment daily, trying whatever appeals to you and your family's lifestyle.

The goal is and should always be to improve your life and your family's health. Hang in there with me. It's time to empty the bathtub once and for all. You deserve the benefits—and most of all, so does your family.

Chapter 2

get ready to detox naturally

Help for just about everything you need to detox and start living a natural life may be as close as your pantry and refrigerator. Many everyday kitchen items, including baking soda, olive oil, and herbs and spices, can double as natural solutions for a host of uses, without any toxic side effects.

Before we dive into the five steps, I want to run through a list of supplies, including cooking utensils, you'll want to have on hand. You may be surprised by how many of these items you already own. You really don't need much to get started, with the exception of some special containers to hold your natural products. I'm not going to list every single ingredient found in the recipes, since you'll be picking and choosing which ones to make. I'll just give you a list of supplies that will help make your detox and your new natural lifestyle a lot easier. If you want to see the same ingredients and

supplies I use in these recipes (as well as premade safe alternatives), check out the full list at WellnessMama.com/detox-book/.

BASIC COOKING UTENSILS

You'll be cooking up most of the recipes in your kitchen, so you'll want to have enough pots and pans, cooking spoons, baking dishes, muffin tins, and so forth on hand. I don't use the same utensils for food that I use for my natural products, so it helps to get some extra ones that are dedicated only to home remedies, natural cosmetics, and natural household cleaners.

Some of the most necessary utensils include:

Double boiler

Silicone baking mat

Silicone baking cups (for homemade soaps)

Mini-food processor (I picked mine up at a thrift shop)

Strainer or a supply of cheesecloth or gauze

Small muslin bag

Glass mixing bowls, various sizes

CONTAINERS

Just about everything you make will be stored in containers, and there are some special kinds you'll need to buy. You can reuse empty cosmetic jars and containers. Just make sure you wash them out thoroughly. Here's a list of must-have containers:

Glass jars with airtight lids, in various sizes: quart, pint, and 8 ounce (mason jars are my favorite)

Tins, vials, bottles, or small jars (with lids or stoppers) for storing tinctures

Dark-colored dropper bottles

Empty liquid soap dispenser

Old makeup containers

Silicone squeezable tubes

Lotion bar tubes

Spray bottles (preferably glass) in various sizes

ESSENTIAL OILS

As you look through my recipes, you'll find that they incorporate many types of essential oils. Our first and oldest medicine, essential oils have been used for centuries by ancient civilizations in Egypt, India, Greece, and Rome. In India, the Ayurvedic medical tradition has relied on essential oil massage as a healing treatment for centuries.

Today, these concentrated plant compounds hold an important place in the healing arsenal right beside conventional medications and herbal medicine. When used and administered properly, they are effective against many conditions, including the common cold, arthritis, and menopausal symptoms.

As a general rule, look for high-quality essential oils, and buy organic when possible. Find the ones I use at WellnessMama.com/go /essential-oils.

Typically, essential oils can be used in several ways:

1. Topically, either diluted or "neat" (undiluted) on the skin.

2. Aromatically by diffusing them into the air.

3. Internally by ingesting them (I do not recommend using oils in this way. If they are used internally, it should be under the direct guidance of a qualified health professional).

Topical Use

The first, and most common method, is topical application. You can massage the oils onto your skin, usually in a diluted form, or place them in baths. A good example might be lavender oil rubbed directly on an insect bite to stop itching.

When using on the skin, dilution is important. It helps reduce the chance of a negative reaction and also increases the effectiveness by spreading out the application over a bigger area. With oils, more is not better, and a small amount can be more effective than a larger amount. In fact, some essential oils such as ylang ylang and lemongrass can cause a reaction, so you should never apply them undiluted.

In general, the younger the person, the more the oil should be diluted. Personally, I do not use essential oils on babies under age two (many are not considered safe for children this young), and I stick to a 1 percent dilution for kids younger than twelve. I find other remedies easier and safer for children these ages. For adults, I opt for a 2.5 percent dilution and sometimes go as high as 5 percent for muscle soreness or other acute uses. Dilution ratios vary with the oil (see the "Common Uses for Essential Oils" chart on page 20), and you have to experiment.

Inhalation and Aromatherapy

A second use is aromatherapy, the inhalation of the aroma, often after the essential oil or oils are placed in a diffuser or from their simple release into the air. This triggers the "vital essence" of the oil that interacts with our nervous systems, our tissues, and our bloodstreams to produce antiviral, anti-inflammatory, pain-relieving, and antidepressant benefits.

In many cases, inhaling oils can be more effective than topical use, but when oils are used in beauty products, it is still important to follow proper dilution ratios. Using essential oils on your skin also allows a slow-release effect as the oils are absorbed slowly over time. Inhalation provides a much faster dose.

Inhalation through aromatherapy can thus be more effective than topical or internal use and is also much safer. As you'd guess, this means diffusing oils into the air so they are taken in by the lungs in small amounts. Some oils are not considered kid safe, even via inhalation, so I stick to kid-friendly blends for diffusing. Here is just a short list of essential oils that are 100 percent safe for children when diffused or applied topically:

Blue tansy	Helichrysum
Cedarwood	Lavender
Copaiba	Mandarin
Cypress	Neroli
Geranium	Sandalwood
German chamomile	Tea tree

Essential oils are also a fragrant addition to topical homemade products, as well as to household cleaners.

Ingestion

Essential oils may be taken orally, although I don't recommend this without the oversight of a trained medical practitioner as some are dangerous to ingest.

Versatility

Essential oils can also be used around the house to control bugs, purify water and air, banish mold and fungus, and freshen musty odors. They also make great insect repellents. Mosquitoes hate lavender, for example. So a few drops of lavender oil on your skin before going outside can prevent you from being eaten alive.

There are hundreds of essential oils available. Here is a list of some of the oils you'll want to have on hand:

Basil	Lemon
Bergamot	Orange
Clove	Patchouli
Eucalyptus	Peppermint
Lavender	Rosemary

COMMON USES FOR ESSENTIAL OILS

CONDITION	OIL	ADMINISTRATION	BEST CARRIERS	DILUTION
ACNE	Tea tree oil	Topically on affected areas	Apricot kernel or argan oil or aloe vera gel	Add 2 drops per teaspoon of carrier oil or gel.
ALERTNESS	Basil, cinnamon, clove, ginger, peppermint, rosemary, or sage oil	Inhaled with a diffuser or used in bathwater	Water	Add 5 to 10 drops to a warm-water bath, and take deep breaths so the stimulating properties take effect.
ALLERGIES, SEASONAL	Chamomile, eucalyptus, lavender, or rose oil (used alone or blended)	Topically under the nose	Just about any carrier oil	Add 2 to 3 drops to equal parts carrier oil.
CONSTIPATION	Fennel, ginger, or rosemary oil	Topically massaged on the abdomen	Coconut oil	Add 1 drop to 3 or 4 drops warmed coconut oil.
CUTS AND BRUISES	Lavender or tea tree oil	Topically on affected areas	Coconut oil	Add 2 drops per teaspoon of carrier oil or gel.
DEPRESSION	Chamomile, cinnamon, clary sage, clove, lavender, or lemon oil	Inhaled or used in bathwater	Water	Add 5 to 10 drops to a warm-water bath, and take deep breaths so the mood-boosting takes effect.
GUM DISEASE	Tea tree oil	Topically on gums	Water	Mix 5 to 10 drops tea tree oil with 1 cup water, and use as a mouthwash.
HEADACHE	Lavender oil	Topically on temples or inhaled	Rose hip oil	Add 5 to 10 drops to a warm-water bath, and take deep breaths to reduce headache tension.
HIGH BLOOD PRESSURE	Neroli, orange, geranium, or clary sage oil	Topically massaged over entire body	Grapeseed or sweet almond oil	Mix 6 or 7 drops with 2 teaspoons carrier oil.
INSECT BITES	Lavender oil	Used in bathwater	Water	Add 10 drops to a warm-water bath, and soak in the tub for 20 to 30 minutes.

CONDITION	OIL	ADMINISTRATION	BEST CARRIERS	DILUTION
INSOMNIA	Lavender, peppermint, or chamomile oil	Topically, sprayed on pillow, or inhaled	Water	Add 5 to 10 drops to a warm-water bath, and take deep breaths for relaxation.
ITCHING	Peppermint oil	Topically on affected areas	Sweet almond or jojoba oil	Add 2 drops per teaspoon of carrier oil.
MENTAL FATIGUE	Cinnamon oil	Topically on temples	Olive oil	Add 2 drops per teaspoon of carrier oil.
MUSCLE ACHES	Ginger, nutmeg, or rosemary oil	Topically or in bathwater	Grapeseed, olive, or coconut oil	Add 2 drops per teaspoon of carrier oil; add 5 to 10 drops to a warm-water bath.
NAUSEA OR MOTION SICKNESS	Lemon oil or ginger oil	Topically	Coconut oil	Add 2 drops per teaspoon of carrier oil.
RELAXATION FROM STRESS	Chamomile, clary sage, lavender, or lemon oil	Used in bathwater		Add 5 to 10 drops to a warm-water bath, and take deep breaths to reduce tension.
SINUS AND COLD SYMPTOMS	Eucalyptus or rosemary oil	Topically around nose or on chest or inhaled	Coconut oil, water	Add 2 drops per teaspoon of carrier oil. For inhalation, pour 2 cups boiling water in a small bowl, then add 5 to 10 drops essential oil. Lean in until your nose is 12 inches from the bowl and inhale.
SKIN CONDITIONS SUCH AS ECZEMA, PSORIASIS, AND GENERAL IRRITATION	Chamomile oil	Topically	Sweet almond or jojoba oil	Add 2 drops per teaspoon of carrier oil.
SUNBURN	Chamomile and lavender oils (blend)	Topically, sprayed on	Carrot seed oil	Add 2 drops per teaspoon of carrier oil.
TOOTHACHE	Chamomile or clove oil	Topically on the tooth	Coconut oil	Add 2 drops per teaspoon of carrier oil.

OTHER OILS

Homemade creams and lotions are a simple mixture of oil, wax, and sometimes essential oils. Common cooking oils, like those you probably have in your kitchen right now, serve as the main moisturizing basis for many of my homemade cosmetics. You'll want to stock your kitchen with the following:

Castor oil

Coconut oil

Olive oil

Sesame oil

Sunflower oil

WAXES

My natural beauty recipes also incorporate cosmetic waxes. The best to use is beeswax. It's a natural emulsifier (which helps bind other ingredients together) that's full of nutrients for your skin. Some recipes call for emulsifying wax, which has slightly different properties from beeswax. A good source for purchasing both is Amazon.

CLAYS

Clays are wonderful for my deep-cleansing masks, because they have the ability to extract toxins and other impurities from the skin. You can thus effectively treat pimples, insect bites or stings, and poison ivy and oak by using clays. They also dry the skin slightly; if your skin is oily, clay makes an effective deep-cleaning mask.

Here's a list of clays I use in my recipes:

Bentonite Clay. Composed of aged volcanic ash, bentonite clay can be used externally as a clay poultice or mud pack and also in the bath and in skin care recipes.

French Green Clay. Also derived from curative volcanic ashes, French green clay draws out impurities and toxins from the skin when used as a mask. It also tones and tightens the skin while stimulating circulation.

Fuller's Earth Clay. This is a type of clay that contains various minerals, including magnesium, quartz, silica, iron, and calcium. It is widely used as a skin-lightening agent and a treatment for oily skin.

Kaolin Clay. You find this clay in facial and skin products, body powders, deodorants, and scrubs. It is perfect for sensitive skin and often used as a base in mineral makeup.

Redmond Clay. This natural clay is highly versatile and is used in facial masks, deodorants, and body powders.

White Cosmetic Clay. A very fine and light clay, this substance has natural absorbency properties. It is used in virtually all powdered and dry cosmetics and a number of wet cosmetics, including soaps, scrubs, deodorants, facial powders, and masks.

MISCELLANEOUS

You should have the following on hand too (if you don't already!):

Apple cider vinegar

Arrowroot or organic cornstarch

Baking soda

Borax

Calcium carbonate powder

Cloth baby wipes (or old scraps of cloth)

Cocoa powder, organic

Distilled water

Dr. Bronner's Original Soap & Sal Suds

Epsom salts

Hydrogen peroxide

Liquid castile soap

Mica powder in color of choice (I use bronze and gold)

Soap nuts

Vodka or rum

Glycerites (alcohol-free herbal tinctures that use vegetable glycerin to extract the medicinal constituents and flavor from an herb)

Washing soda

White vinegar

Witch hazel

Xylitol, finely ground

Zinc oxide powder

2 dozen or more huck towels

1 dozen microfiber cloths

3 or 4 dozen cloth napkins

Other assorted clean cloths, including cut-up old shirts, old cloth diapers/inserts, or old socks (for younger kids to use in cleaning and polishing)

THE BEST "SUPPLY" OF ALL

Most people ask me, "Why would you make so much of your own stuff when you can go to the grocery store and pick from a great selection of products?"

The obvious answer is because of my commitment to natural living. Plus, I like the feeling of independence in learning how to make things on my own. Because of the easy access to all of these products, it's not as common for people to know the basics behind DIY household products. I love the feeling of keeping this knowledge alive, at least in my own home. In the long run, I can really save time and money by not having to run to the store for cosmetics, ointments, pills, cleaning supplies, and other things. Isn't the best of anything usually homemade?

As you go into this, know that you're going to have fun. "Fun" is the greatest supply of all. You can get creative and enjoy the process of discovery. When you get ready to do these, by all means let the kids pitch in. Mine are always eager to help and see the final product.

Going "natural" will give you a sense of satisfaction that you're doing something healthful for yourself, your family, and the environment—you'll even find new motivation to improve all aspects of your life, for the rest of your life.

So let's get started!

the steps

STEP 1: *give your body a new start*

Do you sometimes feel like you're dragging behind instead of being proactive? Do you wish you could think more clearly? Are ailments like constipation, skin problems, fatigue, or allergies interfering with your life?

Many of these symptoms are a result of toxic overload from chemicals in the foods you may be eating. Our bodies aren't designed to process or get rid of this multitude of toxins. And because most chemicals are largely indestructible, when we breathe, absorb, and ingest them—even in tiny amounts—they can build up in our bodies over time. The solution is to detox nutritionally.

In Step 1, you'll learn about foods that support your body's own natural detoxification systems and immune defenses—and how to plan healthful detoxifying meals for you and your family. Changes such as eating organic food (perhaps even growing your own), taking quality supplements, and making your own natural medicines can drastically improve your health and the health of your family. So let's get started. Welcome to Step 1!

Chapter 3

detox with real food

To boost health and rejuvenate yourself, your first move must be to overhaul your diet. The major diseases that plague us today—cancer, stroke, heart disease, diabetes, obesity, and dementia—all have one thing in common: poor diet. Most health experts agree that the best way to slash your odds of getting these diseases is to enjoy more fruits and vegetables and shun processed foods and meats.

When you eat whole natural foods, such as fresh fruits and vegetables, and quality proteins, you're supplying your body with the vitamins, minerals, antioxidants, phytochemicals, enzymes, fiber, amino acids, and nutrition required to prevent all these diseases. All of these nutrients help our bodies self-heal and renew daily. That's why we must eat real food.

Just what is "real" food? I define it as any food in its unprocessed state as created by nature. And usually it's a single-ingredient food too, such as an apple, a piece of salmon, or a serving of spinach. Once you begin to eat more real food, your health and energy levels will improve so much that you'll never want to return to processed food.

THE WELLNESS MAMA FOOD DETOX

I'm not here to tell you to "cleanse" or pick up a single carton of green juice. Instead, I'm going to recommend that you kick out certain foods from your diet—and do so gradually—replacing them with healthful real food.

DITCH THESE FOODS

Bad Vegetable Oils and Fats

Certain fats and oils should be avoided completely. They are chemically processed, high in empty calories, and made with genetically mod-ified grains. What's more, they provoke chronic inflammation in the body, which damages cells, tissues, and organs and leads to life-shortening diseases such as heart disease, stroke, diabetes, cancer, and dementia. The unhealthful ones to avoid or limit are:

Any fake butter or vegetable oil products

Canola oil	Margarine
Corn oil	Peanut oil
Cottonseed oil	Safflower oil
Grapeseed oil	Shortening
I Can't Believe It's Not Butter (you'd better believe it's not!)	Smart Balance (not a smart idea!)
	Soybean oil
	Sunflower oil

"Vegetable" Oil

It is fairly easy to avoid these culprits but not so easy to avoid all the foods they are in. Read the labels of many processed foods, and you will find at least one of these bad fats in them; if a label says "partially hydrogenated corn/soybean/etc. oil" or "may contain soybean or canola oil," you should avoid the product. The following foods, in particular, often contain one of the above unhealthful oils:

Artificial cheeses	Sauces
Chips	Snack foods
Cookies	Store-bought condiments
Crackers	
Mayonnaise	Store-bought nuts
Salad dressings	

Most Sugar

Sugar in any form has no redeeming qualities. It contains no nutrients, no protein, no health-ful fats, and no enzymes. Too much sugar in our diets is responsible for a laundry list of health problems, from obesity, heart disease, and diabetes to behavior problems in kids. Here is a partial list of sugars and sweeteners to avoid:

Agave syrup	Dextrose
All artificial sweeteners, including sucralose and aspartame	Fructose
	Glucose
	High-fructose corn syrup
Brown sugar	
Cane sugar	Sugar alcohols
Corn syrup	Table sugar
	Turbinado sugar

Wheat and Wheat Products

High-wheat diets are implicated in many modern-day health problems, including osteo-porosis, autoimmune diseases, type 2 diabetes, and heart disease. Here are some reasons to avoid wheat:

- It is loaded with phytate, an "antinutrient" that blocks the body from absorbing health-promoting minerals such as zinc, iron, and bone-building calcium.

- It is high in carbohydrates, which in excess can contribute to weight gain. Wheat is also a high-glycemic food; it raises blood sugar and insulin, setting the stage for type 2 diabetes.

- It is high in lectins, such as wheat germ ag-glutinin. This substance triggers inflammation and makes the gut permeable (known as leaky gut syndrome). It can also upset the balance of good and bad bacteria in the gut.

- It is found in gluten, a hard-to-digest protein that in susceptible people leads to celiac disease or gluten sensitivity, which causes very uncomfortable digestive symptoms.

Unhealthful Proteins

Protein is a critical nutrient for good health, but many of the protein sources in the modern diet contain toxins, hormones, antibiotics, and other unhealthful chemicals because of the way cows, poultry, and fish are raised. These are some of the worst offenders:

Conventionally raised beef and organ meats

Conventionally raised chickens and eggs

Farmed seafood

Non-fermented soy (interferes with thyroid function and therefore metabolism)

Nuts cooked in hydrogenated vegetable oils (most of them!)

Sweetened or processed dairy sources

DETOX WITH THESE FOODS

Vegetables and Fruits

Making dietary changes means learning new recipes, new foods, and new habits. It can be intimidating and even scary to change what we're used to. The key is to go step-by-step and keep a positive focus on all of the healthful, delicious, amazing foods nature offers us.

Let's talk about what is always a good choice and will never be a diet "fad." You guessed it: fruits and vegetables—lots of them!

They are the most important food groups for a healthful detoxifying diet. Vegetables and fruits are superior for health. Scientific evidence indicates an association between a high intake of fruits and vegetables and reduced risk of chronic disease—for at least three vital reasons: (1) Vegetables and fruit are rich in a variety of nutrients, including vitamins, trace minerals, antioxidants, phytochemicals, and dietary fiber. (2) Antioxidants and phytochemicals, in particular, activate "detoxification enzymes," natural substances in the body that filter the blood and aid the liver in eliminating toxins. (3) These foods stimulate your immune system, prevent abnormal blood clotting, reduce blood pressure, and generally protect against chronic diseases.

These vegetables and fruits are superstars at detoxification:

Artichokes. Packed with antioxidants, including liver-supportive silymarin, artichokes are also abundant in vitamin C and rich in fiber to keep your system regular.

Avocados. Technically a fruit, avocados are high in fat but mostly the monounsaturated kind, which has been shown to reduce bad LDL cholesterol and promote good HDL cholesterol. Avocados also boast anti-inflammatory nutrients, including omega-3s, antioxidants, and phytosterols, and because they're fiber superstars, they support healthful digestion and detoxification.

Beets and Beet Greens. The skin and flesh of this fibrous root vegetable contain betalains, which boost the activity of detoxification enzymes, according to a 2013 study published in the *British Journal of Nutrition*. The researchers found that betanin protects the liver—the body's main organ of detoxification—and helps prevent cancer. And the greens are a gold mine of minerals and vitamins.

Blueberries. This summer superberry is packed with anthocyanins, the plant pigment responsible for the berry's dark blue hue. Mounds of research link blueberries to greater brainpower and heart health. Blueberries are also low in sugar compared to some other fruits.

Brassica Vegetables. These include broccoli, Brussels sprouts, cauliflower, and cabbage. A growing body of research has found that brassica vegetables protect against many forms of cancer, including tumors of the stomach, pancreas, esophagus, lung, oral cavity and pharynx, endometrium, breast, ovaries, prostate, and colon. Brassica vegetables are also high in phytochemicals, naturally occurring substances in plant foods. These nutrients prevent cell damage, activate detoxification enzymes, stimulate your immune system, and decrease the risk of many cancers.

Spinach. Eating lots of dark leafy greens is key for a healthful diet and particularly imperative for detoxification. Greens such as spinach and kale, full of antioxidants, are thought to have anticancer and detoxification properties, according to a study in *PeerJ* published in 2016. The report mentions that one of the key detoxifying components in these veggies is chlorophyll, which gives these foods their green color. Spinach in particular boasts more than a dozen disease-fighting antioxidants called flavonoids.

Probiotic/Fermented Vegetables

Before I started eating real food, fermented foods like sauerkraut, plain yogurt, and kombucha were not even on my radar. They tasted and smelled too strong to me, and I had no interest in eating them.

Fast-forward a couple years, and I decided to experiment with these foods. I actually started to enjoy them—even crave them from time to time. Now they are a family staple.

Fermented foods are produced or preserved by microorganisms, such as yeast or bacteria. During fermentation, the natural sugars are converted into acids, gases, or alcohol (depending on the food). This process preserves the food and creates beneficial enzymes, B vitamins, omega-3 fatty acids, and various strains of probiotics.

Specific benefits of fermented foods include the following:

Probiotics. Fermented foods and beverages such as yogurt and kefir introduce good bacteria into your digestive system and help the balance of bacteria in your gut. Probiotics also help slow or reverse some diseases, improve digestion, aid in weight loss, and boost immunity.

Improved Food Absorption. The proper balance of bacteria in your gut helps you absorb more of the nutrients in the foods you eat. Pair this with a healthful real-foods diet and your body will take in many more nutrients from food.

Food Preservation. Fermented foods do not go to waste as easily as other foods. You can store these foods longer but without losing the nutrients.

Worth singling out here is sauerkraut, a powerful detox food. Not only does it supply probiotics, it is made solely from cabbage. Cabbage contains compounds known as glucosinolates, which rev up detoxification enzymes and help protect liver cells and other organs, according to an article published in the *Journal of Nutrition* in 2005 and several other studies found in the scientific literature.

Good Proteins

Protein provides the building blocks for muscle and other tissues, repairs and regenerates cells, and boosts mental energy. It also strengthens your immune defenses, transports oxygen and nutrients throughout the body, and produces hormones and enzymes required for great health.

The best sources of protein are organic and humanely raised and free of antibiotics, hormones, dyes, and other toxins. Choose from the following:

Chunk-light (not albacore) tuna or sardines (in water, not vegetable or soybean oil!)

Free-range pastured chickens and eggs

Grass-fed beef and beef organ meats

Raw organic nuts and seeds (soaked overnight and dried) and their butters and milks

Whole full-fat organic plain yogurts

Wild game like deer, elk, turkey, etc.

Wild-caught salmon and other fish

Wild-caught shrimp and lobster

Good Fats

To detox, you're excluding many bad fats from your diet. You won't miss a single one, however. There are so many other wonderful and healthful fats that taste great and support great health:

Avocados and avocado oil	Nuts
	Olive oil
Butter	Organic cream
Coconut oil	Palm oil
Flaxseed oil	Walnut oil
Macadamia nut oil	

Moderately Healthful Sweeteners

In moderate servings from time to time, honey and stevia are fine. Honey contains about 53 percent fructose but is completely natural in its raw form and has many health benefits. It is high in disease-fighting antioxidants and works as a natural antibacterial agent. Stevia is made from the very sweet leaf of the South American stevia plant, which is completely safe (in its natural form). It also contains few to no calories. You can even grow stevia in pots on your windowsill and add the leaves to iced tea.

Gluten-Free Grains

If you eat grains, I recommend whole gluten-free varieties, such as buckwheat, millet, amaranth, quinoa, and white basmati rice. Gluten is a protein naturally found in different grains, such as wheat, barley, and rye. Although it has a bad reputation, gluten performs some good duties. It helps bread and bread products rise and stay moist, fresh, and chewy, for example.

However, there has been a surge in the number of people diagnosed with celiac disease, an immune reaction to eating gluten. And there are other people who are sensitive to gluten and get digestive upsets after eating it. We're hearing a lot about this now because gluten is not the same as it was a decade ago. Due to new farming methods, there's more gluten in processed food than ever. Essentially modern farming has blended varieties of wheat to create hybrids that grow faster, yield more crops, and create fluffier bread and grain foods, but these hybrid wheat products are also high in gluten. Our digestive systems just can't handle that much gluten. My take on all this is simply to avoid gluten as much as you can.

If you choose to eat gluten-free grains, I advise rotating them. Eat them moderately, rather than eating just one type every day or even every week. If you eat a food too often, your body could develop an allergy-like reaction to that food. Plus, eating a wide range of foods supplies more nutrients.

I still avoid most grains, especially if they contain gluten. Whenever possible, I use vegetables in place of grains. I make simple substitutes like using cabbage for noodles in spaghetti or sweet potatoes instead of noodles in lasagna. Not only are these substitutes more nutritious, but they also taste delicious.

Try baking with grain-free flours such as coconut flour or almond flour, which are higher in protein and fiber. Cassava flour and plantain flour (sources of resistant starch) are also yummy substitutes.

ALWAYS EAT REAL FOOD, PREFERABLY ORGANIC

Your body prefers to digest real foods. It does not like to digest packaged processed foods that contain additives, enhancers, dyes, and flavors, and so forth. All of these wreak havoc on digestion and overall health.

It's best to purchase unprocessed and organic food, since going organic is one of the easiest ways to avoid toxic threats to your health. Thankfully, organic foods can now be found in most supermarkets.

Does buying organic food mean going bankrupt? Cost is currently the biggest concern about organic foods. Well, if you cut out processed foods and drinks, you'd slice a large chunk off your weekly food bill.

The biggest benefit is the gift of health when you ditch processed foods and choose to eat food that is closer to how nature has presented it. You get ample vitamin and nutrient benefits, tons of energy, and less susceptibility to illness. Eating this way sustains you in the most optimal way possible and ensures a healthy body, mind, and spirit.

5 DETOX BENEFITS OF LEMON WATER IN THE MORNING

To support detoxification, start your day with warm lemon water. It offers five important benefits.

1. HELPS DIGESTION

Drinking any water, especially warm water, first thing in the morning can help flush your digestive system and rehydrate your body. Adding some freshly squeezed lemon juice "spikes" the warm water with nutritional and detoxification benefits.

2. A NATURAL FLUSH

Drinking enough water, especially in the morning, helps make sure that the liver can do its job of detoxifying the body effectively. Lemon juice helps stimulate this process.

3. A LITTLE IMMUNE SYSTEM BOOST

Lemons contain vitamin C, though not a spectacularly high amount (30 to 50 mg per lemon). They also contain potassium, an electrolyte. Drinking lemon water first thing in the morning gives the body a small jolt of these nutrients for an immune boost. Vitamin C is also good for the adrenals (which help the body fight stress) and can therefore help reduce the effects of stress.

4. HAPPIER SKIN

By flushing the body and improving digestion, lemon water can promote cleaner, more glowing skin. The vitamin C in lemons supports collagen production, which helps keep skin firm and healthy.

5. HEALTHFUL WEIGHT

Drinking water, especially lemon water, first thing in the morning may help you control your weight. One reason is that sufficient hydration increases metabolism, according to researchers in Germany. Drinking sufficient water throughout the day supports other good weight-loss habits, including nutrition and exercise.

Chapter 4

take the stress out of meal planning

Good meal planning helps you stick to a real-foods diet. Sure, it's much easier to cook a quick convenience food or head to a restaurant when everyone is hungry and nothing is defrosted, but a little planning can prevent these habits.

If you have kids, let them get involved in the planning as well. This will help them get excited about the healthful foods you're cooking, and they'll be more willing to try them.

Following are tips to help you plan out weekly meals for your family that you can start incorporating in your family's lifestyle.

HAVE A DAILY TEMPLATE

Rather than starting from scratch each week, I have a template of the general types of foods I cook each day of the week and the number of times I use each main food. My weekly template looks like this:

- 1 to 2 stir-fries

- 1 salad

- 1 slow-cooker or soup meal

- 1 fish/seafood meal

- 1 to 2 meals from a different cuisine from around the world

- 1 to 2 prepare-ahead oven meals

I try to use the same type of meat no more than twice in a given week, so I might have two beef meals, two chicken meals, one fish meal, and two pork or egg meals. Here's an example of how we eat through the week at my house; the recipes can be found on my website, WellnessMama.com.

SAMPLE WEEKLY WELLNESS MAMA MENU

It can be tough to break the cereal-and-sandwich mind-set, but a time-saving way to eat healthfully is to make extras of foods and serve the leftovers for lunch (or even breakfast), as this sample menu plan illustrates. Here, lunches are always leftovers or a big salad with lots of veggies and leftover meat. If leftovers are short but you have some frozen premade soup on hand (like tomato soup, roasted garlic soup, or butternut squash soup), you can serve them together.

Additionally, many leftover foods can be added to an omelet for breakfast or put into a salad for lunch. Cold meats or barbecue actually make a delicious breakfast or lunch when served with some veggies or eggs.

Another easy trick is to make salads in mason jars (liquid at the bottom for salads, then meat/toppings, then lettuce). Then the meal can be easily dumped onto a plate and served. Other leftovers can be stored in the same way and easily reheated.

DAY 1
Breakfast: Breakfast Sausage and over-easy eggs with sliced tomatoes

Dinner: Greek Meatballs with Roasted Vegetable Salad

DAY 2
Breakfast: Brainpower Smoothie

Dinner: Baked Salmon with Asparagus

DAY 3
Breakfast: Leftover salmon scrambled with eggs and chopped spinach

Dinner: Moroccan Chicken Stir-Fry with sliced raw vegetables and Homemade Ranch Dressing dip

DAY 4
Breakfast: Almond Flour Pancakes topped with fresh berries, Avocado Egg Bake

Dinner: Crockpot Barbecue Ribs with Sweet Potato Fries and Coleslaw

DAY 5
Breakfast: Cheesy Breakfast Casserole

Dinner: Grilled Chicken Citrus Salad

DAY 6
Breakfast: Caprese Omelet

Dinner: Pakistani Kima with side salad

DAY 7
Breakfast: Breakfast Egg Muffins

Dinner: Fish Taco Salad

FOCUS ON CORE RECIPES

Discover and identify recipes your family enjoys. Then make them your "core" recipes, ones that you'll repeat every few weeks. Try to build up to about twenty of these, and you won't ever be bored with your meals. Each week, use these core meals for five of your dinners. Then try something new for two dinners. If you get really motivated, develop variations on these twenty core meals so that you're using fresh in-season produce. This system helps you save money on food too.

STRETCH YOUR PROTEIN

Protein tends to be the most expensive part of the meal. To cut costs, use less expensive cuts of meat and "stretch" them. That way, you can afford to buy organic and grass-fed meats more often rather than relying on more expensive cuts of conventional meats.

Stretch your protein by using it in stir-fries, soups, and casseroles—but use less protein and more veggies. Seasonal veggies are always less expensive and more nutrient dense. Focus on green veggies that are in season to help keep your budget in line.

If you haven't already, invest in a slow cooker or pressure cooker. This helps make tougher cuts of meat more tender and easier to eat (plus they save time!).

MIX IT UP WITH DIFFERENT FLAVORS

A basic easy stir-fry or casserole can taste completely different just by changing the spices. Add some cumin and chili powder for Mexican flavor or some curry for Indian flavor.

Basil, thyme, oregano, and garlic lend an Italian flavor, while Chinese five-spice powder gives these dishes an Asian flair. I buy dried herbs singly in bulk and mix my own spice blends. Not only does this save money, but it avoids the fillers and additives found in many store-bought spice blends.

One of my dreams is to travel the world and try the different cuisines in each country. Because that isn't possible right now, I try to create the same experience in my kitchen. With a little research and some healthful adjustments, you can create recipes from around the world. You might be surprised to find that your kids enjoy the flavors of Indian or Thai food or that you have a passion for French flavors.

DON'T BE A SHORT-ORDER COOK

The best way to ensure you raise a picky eater is to let your children eat whatever they want and cater to their food preferences.

Want to *not* raise a picky eater? Expose your children to healthful and diverse foods, starting from a young age, and don't make any specific foods just for them. My one-year-old gladly eats curries, cooked vegetables, liver, and avocado because she's never had crackers, toast, chicken nuggets, or juice. Not only is this approach more nutritious for kids, but it will really be a benefit to them in the long run.

We have two basic food rules in our household:

1. The One-Bite Rule. Kids are required to try one bite of everything I've cooked before they can have more of any one food (I only put one bite on their plate at first). This stops the stress

MAKE YOUR OWN BABY FOOD

Moms like me have turned to making their own baby food in an effort to start our babies off healthfully. If you've never considered doing this, it's easier than you think. Benefits include:

- You can control what goes into homemade baby food. Commercial brands might contain additives, preservatives, and pesticides—none of which I want to feed to a baby.

- Homemade is fresher.

- Homemade is cheaper. You save because you aren't paying for the extra packaging, advertising, and profits a company adds into the price of its product.

Here are my personal dos and don'ts for making baby food:

DO try breastfeeding. The most healthful first food for babies is breast milk. Full of fatty acids, antibodies, nutrients, protein, and good fat, it is a truly perfect and complete food for babies. Research also shows that breastfeeding drastically reduces the instance of SIDS (of every eighty-seven deaths from SIDS, only three are breastfed babies). There are benefits to mom too: decreased risk of cancers (breast, ovarian, cervical, endometrial); lower incidence of postpartum depression; and reduced chance of heart disease, stroke, and diabetes. If breastfeeding is not possible, thankfully there are some great organic options for formula.

DON'T start solid food with oatmeal or rice cereal. Cereals will be recommended, particularly iron-fortified rice. Babies do need nutrients like iron at around six months, but is a "fortified" food the best way to go rather than a food that naturally contains iron and other nutrients? No. Fortification indicates that a food is processed; there are better ways to supply your infant with iron and other minerals (see next page). Another reason that rice cereal and other starchy foods aren't the best first choice for baby is that at age four to six months, babies don't make enough of an enzyme called amylase to break down most carbohydrates. This means that starchy foods like rice can irritate a baby's digestive system and lead to discomfort in some infants.

DO feed your baby bone broths. Broth may seem like an odd first food for a baby, but it is a superfood for gut health. It contains nutrients that help "heal and seal" an infant's gut and improve the symptoms of leaky gut. Babies are naturally born with a leaky gut because this allows beneficial antibodies and enzymes from mom's milk to pass into the bloodstream and increase immunity. Eventually, the gut needs to seal so that particles from foods and pathogens don't enter the bloodstream as well. Broth is also a great source of gelatin, amino acids, bioavailable minerals, and other nutrients. Any bone broth recipe will do, or you can purchase organic bone broth online from Amazon or dietary supplement companies.

DO feed meat and liver. After broth, I'll introduce pastured grass-fed high-quality meats and liver that have been lightly cooked and very finely grated to the broth. Meat is a complete source of protein and amino acids, and liver is nature's multivitamin. Even small amounts of these foods will supply the iron and zinc babies need, and these foods are less likely to be allergenic than many other foods.

DO feed mashed banana and avocado. I often mash these into the meat or broth. Bananas are one of the few fruits that contain amylase, making them easier to digest for most babies. Avocado is packed with beneficial fats and another good first fruit or vegetable choice.

DO include butter and other vegetables. Add in grass-fed pastured butter (for the healthful fats and vitamin K2) and other nonstarchy vegetables. I add vegetables one at a time and usually about a week apart. Vegetables have a much higher nutrient content than grains and pose less chance of an allergic response, so I introduce almost all vegetables before any grains, including rice. Commercial baby food doesn't have anywhere near the nutrients of fresh steamed vegetables.

DO be careful about eggs. Eggs can be highly allergenic to infants, even though they are recommended as a first food for babies. Hold off on eggs until your child reaches the toddler stage.

DON'T puree. My kids are adventuresome, independent eaters. One reason is I never pureed baby food. I just made sure that all foods were cut into small enough pieces to prevent choking and were cooked so that they were extremely soft. I'd then just place them on the table for my babies to reach. They loved feeding themselves these little pieces of food. This kept them busy and happy, so I could serve the rest of the family and even eat something myself!

DO keep it clean. Wash your hands and all equipment thoroughly before starting. Choose organic foods. Babies generally prefer one-ingredient meals in the beginning, so keep your meals simple.

that comes from facing a whole plate of a new food. It also reduces food waste.

2. **The No-Thank-You Rule.** If my kids are truly not hungry, they are not required to eat; however, they cannot complain about the food or interrupt the meal with a bad attitude. I'm not a fan of forcing foods on kids or mandating finishing everything on a plate. At the same time, food is first and foremost for nourishment and not being hungry isn't an excuse to complain about the food being served.

Certainly, there are times when my kids are not happy with these rules or the foods they are served, but as with other areas of parenting, sometimes the best option for children is not always the one they enjoy most!

SAVE TIME WITH BATCH COOKING

As a busy mom, I sometimes spend hours in the kitchen each day. As soon as I finish cleaning up from one meal, it's time to prepare the next. The way I get around these time constraints is with "batch cooking." This is simply preparing large batches of meals ahead of time, putting them in containers, and refrigerating or freezing them. As an example, I'll often precook protein like chicken and beef and preroast big trays of vegetables. These can be repurposed and easily made into soups or a quick stir-fry on a busy night. The time it takes to batch-cook saves me hours of meal-prep time later.

I do my batch cooking on Saturdays, when the kids are playing in the backyard with friends, and I have a few hours to spare. It takes a little trial and error to get used to, but once you give it a try, it will become a good habit.

Also, batch cooking helps us stick to our meal plans, because most of the food is already prepped and there really isn't any excuse not to eat it. Far less food goes to waste when you batch-cook.

Organizing your meals around these principles, and selecting healthful organic foods can help you create an optimal diet for your family every day of the week. What's more, these basics will save you time, money, and stress.

Chapter 5

grow your own food

If you want truly pure, organic food in order to detox your body, try growing some of it yourself. Gardening was once a normal part of life for most people, and in almost all parts of the world we still have the ability to grow some of our own food, at least part of the year. However, statistically, many of us don't (especially in the United States). Certainly, as the population has moved away from agriculture and into more urban settings, gardening is not as necessary, and there isn't as much land to garden on, but it is certainly still possible.

I've been home gardening for so long now that I've got it down to a science. Following are my tips and suggestions for getting started, whether you want to grow a few veggies on your windowsill or patio or graduate to becoming a backyard "farmer."

SMALL-SPACE GARDENING

Grow Superfood Sprouts

If you don't have any outdoor space at all, you can still grow a countertop garden in your kitchen with sprouts and microgreens.

Sprouted seeds, beans, and grains are among the richest sources of nutrition you can find. Sprouts are a treasure chest of minerals, enzymes, and amino acids, not to mention antioxidants, which can help to protect against free radicals. They can be easily grown just about anywhere, with minimal equipment. Sprouted beans and grains make nutrients more bioavailable and reduce lectins and phytic acid. I also like sprouting certain seeds and nuts for adding to salads and stir-fries.

Best of all, they take only a few days to

grow. If you've never tried to grow sprouts at home, you are missing out on an easy way to have fresh nutrients year-round.

These are the most common sprouts grown:

Alfalfa	Mung beans
Broccoli	Pumpkin seeds
Chia seeds	Red clover
Lentils	Sunflower seeds

There is equipment specifically designed for sprouting, such as sprouting trays, which make sprouting easier and allow for more growth at once. But if you don't have those, all you really need are:

• A widemouthed quart- or half-gallon-size mason jar

• A sprouting lid or a piece of cheesecloth and a rubber band

• A bowl or box to help the jar stand upside down at an angle

• Organic sprouting seeds—make sure they are specifically labeled "sprouting seeds" and "organic."

Steps for Growing Sprouts

1. Wash your hands well and make sure that all equipment is clean and sterile.

2. Pour one type of seed into the jar. Use about 1 teaspoon small seeds, such as alfalfa or broccoli, or ¼ cup beans and lentils (for a quart-size jar).

3. Cover with 1 cup filtered water and put lid or cheesecloth over the jar.

4. Allow to soak for up to 12 hours. It is often easiest to do this at night and soak overnight.

5. In the morning, strain off the water. This is easily done with a sprouting lid. If you are using a cheesecloth, pour through a fine-mesh strainer and return the seeds to the jar.

6. Rinse the seeds well with filtered water and drain again.

7. Place the jar upside down at a slight angle so that excess water can drain off and air can get in. I find a dish rack or medium bowl is perfect for this.

8. Rinse the sprouts several times a day with filtered water, returning the jar to the tilted position each time.

9. You should see sprouting in a day or two, and most sprouts are ready to harvest in 3 to 7 days.

10. When done sprouting, rinse thoroughly in cool, filtered water, and store in a covered container in the refrigerator for up to a week.

Note: Some seeds (such as walnuts and pecans) do not sprout, and some beans (such as kidney beans) are dangerous and should never be eaten sprouted.

Grow Ultra-Superfood Microgreens

As the name suggests, microgreens are just miniature plants of greens, herbs, or other vegetables. Like sprouts, they are a concentrated nutrient source and packed with beneficial enzymes because of their rapid growth.

Though they are often seen in dishes at restaurants because of their delicate flavor and sophisticated presentation, they are simple to grow on your own and cost very little once you have the supplies. With the right tools, you can have a year-round vegetable source on your kitchen counter.

The most common plants used for growing microgreens are:

Beet	Kale
Buckwheat	Lettuce
Cabbage	Mustard
Chia	Radish
Greens	Spinach
Herbs	Sunflower
Watercress	

MICROGREEN GROWING SUPPLIES

- Sunny spot in a south-facing window or a grow light (optional)

- Organic potting soil to fill the tray

- Shallow tray or planter

- Microgreen seeds (like those listed above)

- Spray bottle, preferably glass

- Warming mat to speed germination (optional)

Steps for Growing Microgreens

1. Find a south-facing window with plenty of sunlight or install an inexpensive grow light. I've found that a grow light mounted under kitchen cabinets works perfectly for growing greens on the counter if you have the space to do it. In warmer months, these can also be easily grown outside.

2. Place an inch of organic potting soil in the bottom of a shallow tray and smooth out evenly. Alternatively, clear an area of your garden for growing microgreens.

3. Scatter seeds over the surface of the soil evenly. Since you are not growing plants to full size, do not worry about spacing the seeds evenly—your sprouts will grow 1 to 2 inches tall and you'll want to harvest as many as possible from each tray. Tip: Soaking the seeds overnight will speed sprouting time but make it more difficult to scatter them.

4. Cover the seeds with a thin layer of soil and spray the surface with clean, filtered water. I use an upcycled glass vinegar bottle with a misting spray top.

5. Place on the warming mat, if using, and in the sunny window or under a grow light.

6. Mist the seeds a couple of times a day to keep the soil evenly moist while waiting for the seeds to germinate.

7. Greens are usually ready to harvest in 2 to 4 weeks, depending on the type of seed used.

8. To grow another crop, either remove the roots and replant or dump the entire tray in the compost and fill with more soil to replant. If you dump in the compost, some straggler seeds usually volunteer and make a crop of their own a few weeks later.

There you go: Growing sprouts and micro-greens on a windowsill or other bright spot in your home is a bona fide simple way to develop a green thumb and become a home gardener without a lot of labor or trouble.

GARDENING IN A SMALL BACKYARD

If you want to further hone your gardening, take it outdoors with small-space backyard gardening. I know many people who are fortunate enough to have a huge backyard with plenty of room to garden, but many of us live in the city and have limited space that barely gets enough sun.

Not to worry. Even in a small backyard or on a porch/patio, some simple vegetables and greens can be grown:

• Beets, radishes, lettuces, and some greens can be grown in light shade to moderate sun and work well in pots on balconies and patios.

• Vines like green beans, peas, and cucumbers can be grown in hanging baskets or in barrels on a deck or patio. Just make sure that container plants get enough sun and water, and that the container has proper drainage.

• Peppers, tomatoes, and beans need more sun (6 to 8 hours a day) for optimal growth.

MY PERSONAL GARDENING TIPS

The size of your garden is determined by the amount of space you have available, but there are great natural containers that fit any yard size—even a small porch!

Natural Containers

There are many preexisting natural containers that will work:

• Bushel baskets

• Old barrels (cut in half)

• Metal drums or planters

• Wooden boxes

• Ceramic pots

Just make sure that any container has adequate drainage and water container plants often.

Square-Foot Garden

Here's one of the first types of backyard gardening I tried when we moved into our first home. The basic concept is to use a 4 × 4-foot raised bed (or several of them) in a very calculated way to maximize the amount of food that can be grown. The 4 × 4-foot bed is divided into sixteen 1-foot squares, and each square is used for one type of plant (based on size).

For instance, you might plant 1 tomato plant in one square, 4 basil plants in another, and 9 spinach plants in another.

To get started, you need:

• A 4 x 4-foot raised-bed kit (or materials to make your own)

• Square-foot gardening grid (optional)

• Soil and sunlight

Raised Beds

An extension of the square-foot garden is a larger raised bed. The square-foot method can actually be used in a larger bed as well to optimize production.

We currently have an 8 × 4-foot raised-bed garden with an additional 4 × 4-foot trilevel bed. The combined structure is enough for us to grow most of the seasonal vegetables for our family. By using companion- and succession-planting methods, we are able to grow food from April to October in our climate.

If you've started eating more real foods, I'm sure you've noticed that it is a little more expensive to serve your family a roasted chicken with some organic vegetables than it is to throw some $1 pasta in a can of $1 sauce (though there is no comparison nutritionally!).

Growing some of your own food, even in small containers on a patio, will let you have fresh organic produce at a fraction of the cost. If you have the room, a medium-to-large garden can produce enough food to feed a family of four to six, especially if you have time to devote to preservation and storage.

STARTING FROM SCRATCH?

It can be a big job to start a garden from scratch, so here are a few of my favorite tips (which I learned the hard way!):

Decide what to grow. In the first year, especially, it can be tough to know how much of each variety to plant. My strategy is to grow foods that (a) we eat the most and (b) are the most expensive to buy organically. For us, this means lots of spinach, strawberries, winter squash, tomatoes (which we can or ferment), herbs, cucumbers (naturally fermented to preserve), blueberries, sweet potatoes, and peppers (usually dried to preserve).

To help figure out how much of each plant to grow and when to plant, check out GrowVeg .com, which offers a free monthlong trial of its garden planning guide, so you can easily visualize how many of each variety to plant.

Start seeds indoors early. Sowing seeds indoors lets you get a head start on the garden and a longer growing season. For plants like tomatoes and peppers, starting them inside is almost necessary for a good growing season.

To make it easy, get small seed-starter trays that can be kept on a kitchen table, windowsill, or counter. There are even organic versions of these starter trays. Start tomatoes and peppers 4 to 6 weeks before you plant them outside, so for us (in the southeast) that means starting early April indoors and transplanting outdoors in mid-May.

To speed up the process, you can pregerminate the seeds in unbleached coffee filters or paper towels in unzipped plastic bags by following these steps:

- Evenly place about 10 seeds with space in between on an unbleached coffee filter.

- Put another coffee filter on top and spray with warm water to dampen.

- Fold the layered filters in half and place in a quart-size or larger plastic bag, but don't zip it.

- Place the bag on a plate and put on top of your refrigerator or in another slightly warm place.

- In 2 to 3 days, you should see tiny sprouts coming from the seeds.

- Use tweezers to place the sprouted seeds in small indoor pots in a sunny window.

Prepare the garden. Figure out how much space you can devote to a garden and plan accordingly. If you just have a few containers on a patio, make sure to get quality soil and use organic fertilizer to maximize production. If you are growing an outdoor garden, consider using raised beds to maximize space and production.

If possible, build raised beds from untreated hardwoods like cedar. For smaller spaces, use the square-foot-gardening system to yield the most production from the smallest space. Even in bigger spaces, multiple square-foot gardens can still maximize production.

Once you have the space for the garden reserved, make sure you have decent soil to work with. Many county extension offices offer soil testing at very inexpensive prices. Getting your soil tested will help you pinpoint what, if anything, you need to add to the soil to make sure your plants grow well.

We tilled in several truckloads of organic compost over the last couple of years. While this was a little pricey up front, it paid off in the long run. Our soil is naturally very acidic dense clay that doesn't drain well. Adding the compost gave us beautiful black soil that produced veggies in abundance last year!

Make the most of your space. You can easily maximize your growing space and often prevent pests with the same methods. To make sure you get the most production from small spaces, practices like intercropping, companion planting, and succession planting can really help.

Try companion planting. Companion planting lets you grow multiple plants that help each other in the same area. A classic example is the Native American custom of planting corn, beans, and squash together. The corn provides a structure for the beans and squash to climb on, and the beans add nitrogen back into the soil to feed the corn and squash.

Another example is planting basil under tomatoes. Besides tasting great together, these two help deter pests from each other and improve each other's growing quality.

Here are my favorite companionable plant combos:

- Basil with tomato to promote growth and keep pests away

- Marigolds throughout the garden to deter pests and reduce nematodes

- Dill with cucumbers

- Catnip, mint, and chamomile with brassicas (cabbage, broccoli, cauliflower, etc.) to deter pests

- Beets under cabbage to maximize space

- Cucumbers with mammoth sunflowers (the sunflowers act as the trellis)

Practice succession planting. Planting a variety of crops in succession will give you more yield from your garden and extend your harvest season, usually spring or fall. For instance, right now, my garden has young cabbage, cauliflower, broccoli, Brussels sprouts, kale, chard, spinach, and lettuce. Once those are harvested, the same beds will become a space for melons or winter squash.

Do vertical gardening. Growing some plants upward rather than letting them sprawl can reduce the amount of space they need and actually increase yield by reducing disease exposure. Trellises and cages are great for tomatoes, cucumbers, vining squash, and others.

CONTROL PESTS NATURALLY, INDOORS AND OUT

I absolutely did not want my home or garden sprayed with any type of commercial pesticides, so I turned to some of the natural pest control ideas I'd used in the garden before and tried new suggestions offered by friends.

Diatomaceous Earth (DE). This is a fine powder made from the fossilized remains of diatoms, a type of algae. It has a very hard shell, is high in silica, and is very sharp, though it is so fine that it doesn't do damage to human tissue or skin. In fact, you can take it internally to get rid of parasites and for its beneficial silica content (helps hair and nail growth). Its sharp/strong structure allows it to puncture the exoskeleton of insects on a microscopic level, causing them to dehydrate and die (while humans and animals are left completely unharmed).

I've found the DE is especially effective for ants, fleas, roaches, and other insects that walk or jump rather than fly. But do avoid inhaling the powder as it can be irritating to the lungs.

When I noticed an invasion, I sprinkled DE liberally on the carpets and in areas where the ants seemed to be entering. Within a day or two, the ant problem resolved, and I just vacuumed up the remaining powder.

Years ago, when we adopted a precious kitten who brought some not-so-precious fleas with her, our apartment became flea infested within days. Thankfully (or unfortunately), we had white carpet, so I just sprinkled DE on the cat and all the floors a couple times a day for a week and the fleas were gone.

Natural Ant Poison. Katie of KitchenStewardship.com suggested this method when I interviewed her on my podcast, and it works quite effectively.

The poison is made with borax and corn syrup (the only thing I'd recommend using corn syrup for). While you wouldn't want to let your children play with or eat it, borax is much less toxic than commercial pesticides.

Katie's method is to mix equal parts borax powder and corn syrup and spread the mixture on an index card. The ants are attracted to the sweetener, eat it, and take it back to their nest. where it poisons them. It will usually take a day or two before you start seeing results.

Natural Fly Traps. Fruit flies can be especially bad some years, and because of their size, they are difficult to trap. Someone at the farmers' market suggested Natural Catch fruit fly traps from Amazon, and they work great. I keep one on the counter near the fruit, and we haven't had trouble with fruit flies since we got them.

Essential Oils Spray. The easiest way to deal with indoor pests is to keep them from coming indoors in the first place. Easier said than done, but I have had good results using a vinegar and essential oils spray on the outside of our doors where flies and ants were coming in.

Mix 2 cups water with 1 cup white vinegar, 50 drops peppermint essential oil, 20 drops basil essential oil, and 20 drops lemon essential oil. It doesn't smell bad and seemed to repel the insects.

Fresh Basil Leaf. I like this natural pest control solution because it has a dual purpose. Fresh basil leaves seem to repel flies effectively, and I love the flavor of basil (pesto, anyone?). I potted some fresh basil plants and placed them near each of our doors. It seemed to cut down on the insect invasion, and we now have an almost endless supply of fresh basil leaves for caprese salads and other recipes.

Even if you decide to grow a few herbs on your windowsill, sprout some seeds, or do a little container gardening, you're officially a gardener—with all the benefits that go with it.

Chapter 6

make your own medicine

Food and herbs have been used for healing since ancient times. In fact, many conventional medicines we use today are derived from plants. White willow bark was the original source of aspirin, and Taxol, a cancer drug, is made from the Pacific yew tree.

Over the years, I've learned to make a wide range of remedies from foods and herbs right in my own kitchen for many minor ailments, including colds, digestive problems, and skin irritations. They're not only inexpensive but also very easy to make, and you don't have to be a certified herbalist to get started!

In general, my family is very healthy, and we use very few pharmaceuticals, thanks to our natural lifestyle and the fact that I make most of my own medicines. Though homemade medicines may not be right for everyone's lifestyle, I've found the natural approach to be health enhancing, empowering, inexpensive,

and safe. With a little knowledge about how to use herbs, I think you'll find making homemade remedies both fun and rewarding. Remember, these remedies are not meant to be a substitute for medical attention but as a supplement or for use in minor cases where professional medical attention isn't necessary.

Following is an overview of the various types of herbal remedies you can make; you can find numerous recipes in Chapter 19.

HERBAL SYRUPS AND HONEYS

Herbal syrups are a great way to get the benefits of medicinal herbs. Kids love syrups and usually take them willingly.

Honey is a great base for an herbal syrup, especially when combined with a little salt. This remedy actually came indirectly from my grandmother who told me that kids sleep better when you give them something sweet and salty at night. Her theory was that it helped regulate blood sugar. Turns out, there may be some scientific backing to this decades-old idea.

Salt can help lower levels of the stress hormone cortisol and balance blood sugar levels, which is what you want at night for restful sleep. Natural sugars elevate insulin slightly, which in turn lowers cortisol (this is one reason my doctor suggests consuming carbohydrates at night and not in the morning). Carbohydrates of any kind may also help tryptophan, a sleep-inducing amino acid, cross the blood-brain barrier and improve melatonin production. Melatonin is a hormone involved in regulating sleep.

Honey by itself is an effective cough soother. In fact, I've heard of doctors recommending a spoonful of honey to children (over a year old) for cough. To honey, you can add ginger, a natural anti-inflammatory with expectorant action.

A good partner for honey is the herb chamomile. It soothes muscles, relieves throat tickles, and promotes restful sleep. Other accompaniments are marshmallow root, which coats and soothes the throat; and cinnamon, which helps boost the immune system and improves taste.

My all-time-favorite home remedy to treat the symptoms of more serious colds, even the flu, is elderberries and elderberry syrup. Naturally high in vitamins A, B, and C, the dried berries can be used to make a variety of remedies, especially when made into a syrup.

Elderberries are near-wonder foods. In fact:

Dr. Madeleine Mumcuoglu, of Hadassah-Hebrew University in Israel, found that elderberry dis-arms the enzyme viruses use to penetrate healthy cells in the lining of the nose and throat. Taken before infection, it prevents infection. Taken after infection, it prevents spread of the virus through the respiratory tract. In a clinical trial, 20 percent of study subjects reported significant improvement within 24 hours, 70 percent by 48 hours, and 90 percent claimed complete cure in three days. In contrast, subjects receiving the placebo required 6 days to recover. (Journal of Alternative and Complementary Medicine 1 [Winter 1995]: 361–69).

My recipe uses homemade elderberry concentrate with synergistic herbs like cinnamon and ginger, plus raw honey for an extra immune boost. If you can't/don't use honey, see the substitution suggestions below the recipe (page 124).

Several natural elderberry syrups are available at health stores or online, but the cost is usually around $15 or more for 4 to 8 ounces. My recipe makes 16 ounces for less than $10 and kids love the taste.

HERBAL TEAS

Herbal teas are the easiest way to dip your toes into homemade herbal medicine. They're a gentle way to get the benefit of herbs and are one of the quickest natural remedies to make. I always keep herbs on hand so I can blend teas, tinctures, and other remedies. Also, herbal teas are a great first remedy to teach children. They are easy to mix and make and a fun way to learn the benefits of herbs. I have a great assortment of herbal tea recipes for you in Chapter 19.

HERB-INFUSED OIL BLENDS

Infused oils are a must to prepare, because they form the base of homemade lotions, salves, and other skin remedies. Most are for external use only. I make these oils ahead of time and have them on hand so I can make remedies as I need them.

To infuse oils, place $1/3$ cup needed herbs in a jar with 2 cups carrier oil (such as olive, almond, or avocado oil). Let it rest for 4 to 6 weeks, then strain the needed amount for the recipe. Alternatively, place herbs and oil in the top of a double boiler and simmer on low for 3 to 4 hours, until oil takes on color and smell of herb. Strain and use in salve recipe. You can make an oil stronger by adding more herb in this step and weaker by using less.

TINCTURES

A tincture is the concentrated liquid form of an herb. It preserves and concentrates the healing properties of the herb, making them more effective and longer lasting. In fact, alcohol-based tinctures have a shelf life of several years. I keep several tinctures on hand for my kids, because they can be used externally, even on small children for relief from common problems.

What's more, alcohol tinctures are good for extracting these beneficial parts of a plant: alkaloids (some), glycosides, volatile oils, waxes, resins, fats, some tannins, balsam, sugars, and vitamins.

Store-bought tinctures tend to be expensive, so I encourage you to try making your own. This can be done in a matter of minutes. You need only a few supplies:

- Pint-size mason jar with tight-fitting lid

- Consumable alcohol like vodka or rum—at least 80 proof (or apple cider vinegar or food-grade vegetable glycerine)

- Herbs of your choice

To make a tincture, select which herbs you plan to use. Almost any herb will work, but research it first to make sure it is safe for use for your specific case (see the Become Your Own Herbalist chart on page 52 for some common herbs and their benefits). Check with a doctor prior to using any herb if you have a health condition.

Fill a jar one-third to one-half full with dried herbs. A half-full jar makes a stronger tincture. Do not pack down the herbs. Pour in just enough boiling water to dampen. (This step is optional but helps to draw out the beneficial properties of the herbs.) Fill the rest of the jar with food grade alcohol and stir with a clean spoon.

Cap the jar tightly and let rest for 3 to 6 weeks in a cool, dry place, shaking daily.

Pour through a strainer into small glass jars or colored dropper bottles. Discard the solids. Cap tightly and store in a cool, dry place for up to 6 months.

How to Use Herbal Tinctures

The standard adult dose is $1/2$ to 1 teaspoon up to three times a day as needed depending on the herb. Kids usually get $1/4$ to $1/3$ of the adult dose. For children, pregnant women, or those not wanting to consume alcohol, it can be poured into a hot liquid like tea to evaporate the alcohol before consuming.

HERBAL POULTICES

A poultice is basically a paste made of herbs, clays, activated charcoal, salts, or other beneficial substances that are wrapped in a piece of cloth and placed on the skin. Often, a waterproof layer of plastic or waterproof cloth is added over the poultice, and the poultice is left on for several hours at a time and changed several times a day.

This can be done with fresh or dried herbs or other beneficial substances. The benefit is that the body gets constant contact with all parts of the herb or plant for an extended period of time. Poultices are often used to help boils, burns, splinters, infections, and other skin problems. Some poultices can even be used externally to help internal problems (after seeing a medical professional!).The herb is made into a thick paste with hot or cold water. Hot water is usually used for poultices that will draw out or remove an abscess, while cold water is used in poultices to treat inflammation.

Traditionally, a fresh or dried herb is ground with a mortar and pestle and mixed with water to form the paste. These days, a blender or mini–food processor can also be used to smash the herb. Ground dried herbs can also be used.

First I smash the herbs, and then I pour a tiny amount of really hot water over them to help extract the beneficial properties. I then let them cool to the desired temperature before applying to the skin.

The thick paste can be placed directly on the skin or wrapped between two layers of clean cloth before applying (depending on the herb). Cheesecloth or thin, organic cotton are great choices for this, but it is important to have a cloth that won't absorb too much liquid or that is too thick to let the herbs come in indirect contact with the skin.

When I used a poultice for a burn on my wrist, I wrapped the herbs between two layers of cheesecloth and placed it directly over the burn. I then wrapped it with plastic wrap to keep it on the skin.

When our son was bitten by a spider, I covered a poultice with some waterproof gauze and taped it onto the skin since it was on his upper leg and there was no easy way to wrap it completely around his leg. The specifics will change based on the remedy being used, but the basic method is the same: thick paste, inside cloth, and placed on wound.

HERBAL SALVES

A salve is basically a thick ointment applied directly to the skin. I make herbal salves with herbal-infused oils, thickened with beeswax pastilles. These salves can treat bites, stings, scrapes, cuts, bruises, and other conditions.

I start by selecting the oil for the salve. The infused oil I use depends on the purpose of the salve. It is preferable to have the oil made prior to preparing the salve.

The shelf life of most homemade salves is a year or two. The salve will eventually turn rancid if not used fast enough. To better preserve your salves, keep them in opaque containers in a cool room or in the refrigerator. Vitamin E oil, or rosemary, oregano, tea tree, eucalyptus, lavender, and thyme essential oils, can be added as additional preservatives.

BECOME YOUR OWN HERBALIST

The list below is a roundup of useful safe herbs and other plants organized by the problems they treat. My recipes use all these herbs. Bear in mind that herbal remedies are not miracle cures. And in general, remember that many herbs shouldn't be taken by children or if you're pregnant or nursing unless you get your physician's okay. It's also a good idea to inform your doctor of all the medications and supplements you take, including herbs.

HERB	USED FOR	FORMS
ALOE	Burns, sunburn, skin irritations	Gel from aloe leaves applied topically
ARNICA	Bruises	Infused oil
BLACK WALNUT POWDER	Fungus and ringworm (external)	Salve applied topically
CALENDULA	Skin rejuvenation	Infused oil
CATNIP	Sleeplessness	Tea, salve applied topically
CHAMOMILE	Digestive upsets, improved sleep; baby lotion (external)	Teas, tinctures, and topical salves
CINNAMON	Coughs, indigestion, gas	Syrup
CLARY SAGE	Hormone balancing (external)	Salve applied topically
CRANBERRY	Urinary tract infections	Juice, tea
DANDELION	Detoxification, digestive upsets; eczema (external)	Tea, tincture, poultice applied topically for eczema
ECHINACEA	Colds, flu, immune-system booster; antibiotic (external)	Tea, tincture, salve applied topically as an antibiotic
ELDERBERRY	Colds, sore throat, flu; hemorrhoids (external)	Syrup, poultice applied externally
EUCALYPTUS	Nasal congestion	Infused oil, salve applied topically
FENNEL SEEDS	Digestive upsets	Tea
FEVERFEW	Headaches	Tea, tincture
GARLIC AND ONIONS	Immune-system booster, antibacterial, warts (external)	Syrup, salad dressing, salve applied topically; poultice applied externally for warts

HERB	USED FOR	FORMS
GINGER	Nausea, digestive upsets, anti-inflammatory	Tea
GOLDENSEAL	Antibiotic (external)	Salve applied topically as an antibiotic
LAVENDER	Cuts, burns, sleeplessness, immune-system booster; anti-aging (external)	Syrup, salve applied topically
LEMON BALM	Anxiety, sleeplessness	Tea
MARSHMALLOW ROOT	Colds, sore throat	Tea, syrup
MINT	Digestive upsets, sleeplessness, sore muscles (external), cracked heel (external)	Tea, salve applied topically
PLANTAIN LEAF	Digestive upsets; cuts, scrapes, and bites (external), as well as eczema (external)	Tincture, infused oil, applied topically; poultice applied externally for eczema
RED RASPBERRY	Hormone balancing	Tea
ROSEMARY	Circulatory problems, immune-system booster; scalp health and hair growth (external)	Tea, infused oil applied topically to scalp, salve
SAGE	Sore throat	Mixture of sage and water used as a gargle
SLIPPERY ELM	Sore joints	Poultice
ST. JOHN'S WORT	Depression, anxiety; bruises and skin irritations (external)	Tea, tincture; infused oil applied topically
THYME	Sore throat	Tea, tincture
TURMERIC	Anti-inflammatory, joint pain	Tea, cooking additive
VALERIAN	Anxiety, sleeplessness	Tea, tincture, salve applied topically
WHITE WILLOW BARK	Headache, other aches	Tea, tincture

HEALING CLAYS

Healing clays have been employed for centuries by various cultures around the world—and there are dozens of other ways to use them. Even animals instinctively know the benefits of certain clays and earth substances and can sometimes be seen eating dirt or clays to rid the body of toxins or illnesses.

There are many types of healing clays. One of the best known and most powerful healing clay is bentonite or montmorillonite clay. Bentonite can be used externally as a clay poultice, mud pack, or in the bath and in skin care recipes. A good-quality bentonite should be a gray or cream color, and anything bordering "pure white" is suspect. It has a very fine, velveteen feel and is odorless and nonstaining. It can be found in sodium bentonite or calcium bentonite form. The name comes from the largest-known deposit of bentonite clay, which is located in Fort Benton, Montana.

Like other clays, bentonite clay carries a strong negative charge that bonds to the positive charge in many toxins. When it comes in contact with a chemical or harmful substance, the clay binds to and releases its minerals for the body to use. Bentonite also boosts the amount of oxygen to cells by extracting excess hydrogen and thus allowing the cells to replace it with oxygen instead.

Healing clays like bentonite also have a high concentration of minerals, including silica, calcium, magnesium, sodium, iron, and potassium.

Noted natural medicine expert Dr. Weston A. Price reported in his book *Nutrition and Physical Degeneration* that several Native cultures, including those in the Andes, Central Africa, and Australia, consumed clays in various ways, most often by carrying balls of dried clay in their bags and dissolving a small amount of the clay in water with meals to prevent poisoning from any toxins present.

I've used a teaspoon of bentonite clay in water for digestive disturbances such as acid reflux, constipation, bloating, gas, and so forth. It also eases skin and allergy issues and can be used in oral health remedies. Check with a doctor before ingesting clay or any other substance, especially if you are on medication.

Caveat: Do not let healing clays like bentonite come into contact with anything metal; this reduces their effectiveness. I mix the clay with water in a glass jar with a plastic lid, and shake it well.

If you take it internally, for best results do not take within an hour of food and do not take within two hours of medications or supplements because it might reduce their effectiveness. Check with your doctor before using clays if you have any medical concerns.

Ease into the whole process of making your medicines. Don't try to learn everything at once. Stick with an herb or two that works for you, or experiment with a couple of recipes at first. Do this and you're well on your way to becoming a home herbalist!

STEP 2: *enhance your beauty regimen*

I don't know of a woman or man alive who doesn't want to look their best, and there are tens of thousands of products ready to help. The problem is, though, that cosmetics and beauty products are overformulated with lots of chemicals. All these chemicals are soaked up by the skin, which is the largest organ in our bodies. Unknowingly, we're absorbing lots of toxins directly into our bodies. This can have a major impact on the body's ability to function as designed. Switching from certain personal care products to natural alternatives is the answer, and there's nothing more natural than making your own skin creams, hair care treatments, bath products, and more. Welcome to Step 2!

Chapter 7

your face: keep it soft and ageless

A daily skin care regimen is vital to achieving and maintaining a youthful glow—especially when you use chemical-free beauty products you make yourself. The regimen I put forth in this chapter will detox and revitalize your skin, keeping it soft and preventing wrinkles. You can find all my recipes in Chapter 19.

WASH YOUR FACE

A good beauty routine for your face starts with cleansing. The most effective cleansing agent for your face is a natural oil. Though it sounds crazy at first, it makes a lot of sense. The basic idea of oil cleansing is to use natural oils in specific combinations to cleanse the skin and naturally balance the skin's own oils. This method produces much more nourished and moisturized skin than traditional soap and detergent-based facial cleansers ever will.

The most common oils used are castor oil and olive oil, though any natural oil can work effectively. Castor oil is naturally astringent, so it helps pull impurities from the skin, making it ideal for oily or combination skin (and even for dry skin in lesser amounts). Castor oil should never be used undiluted on the skin, and I always add at least twice the amount of another oil as castor oil when making an oil blend.

My favorite other oil to use is olive oil, although sunflower, safflower, and coconut oils also work great.

If you are new to oil cleansing, it may take a couple of tries to figure out what blend of oils works best for you. Personally, I use a mix that is 3 parts olive oil to 1 part castor or hazelnut oil, and it is perfect for my skin. But one of these ratios might work better for your skin type:

- Oily skin: 1 part castor oil or hazelnut oil to 2 parts olive, sunflower, or other oil

- Combination skin: 1 part castor or hazelnut oil to 3 parts olive, sunflower, or other oil

- Dry skin: All nourishing oils like olive oil or a very small amount of castor oil or hazelnut oil added to the nourishing oils.

To find out the best blend for you, start with the suggested amounts above for your skin type and adjust if needed. When I started to oil-cleanse, I mixed up very small batches (1 teaspoon castor oil to 2 teaspoons olive oil) until I figured out the right blend for me.

I've also found that even pure coconut oil works great once your skin has adjusted, though it can be drying on some skin types. One of my friends uses a half-and-half mix of coconut oil and olive oil blended in a blender to create a cream, and this works perfectly for her.

Steps for Oil Cleansing

1. In your shower or at the bathroom sink, pour a small amount of the oil blend (about the size of a quarter) into your hand and massage into the skin on your dry face.

2. Use smooth circular strokes. Let this be a gentle facial massage, too. Massage for at least a minute (2 minutes is better) or until you are sure that the oil has saturated your skin. This will also remove makeup very effectively, so there is no need to take off your makeup first. You can even leave the oil on the skin for up to 10 minutes to deep clean your pores.

3. Place a clean washcloth under very hot tap water (or shower water) until it is completely soaked and quickly wring it out. Open it and place over your face. This will create steam against the skin to remove the oils and any impurities in the skin. Leave the washcloth on for about 1 minute, or until it cools.

4. Repeat if needed with the other side of the washcloth. Use the corners of the washcloth to gently remove any remaining oil. There will still be a thin layer of oil on your skin, but this is beneficial.

Typically, you won't need any moisturizer after the adjustment period. If you still have dry skin, try reducing the amount of oil and use a tiny bit of organic lotion to moisturize your skin.

It's normal for it to take a week or so for skin to adjust, and you may even see more oily skin or more breakouts during this time as impurities leave your skin. If you can, resist the urge to use harsh soaps or facial cleansers during this time, because they will make the adjustment period longer.

Also important: If you oil-cleanse in the shower, make sure to clean your shower floor regularly so it doesn't get slippery.

Remove Eye Makeup

Oil cleansing will take off your facial makeup, but you need to make sure that you remove eye makeup as well. I admit, I was always leery of mascara remover, because it seemed dangerous to put something like that close to my eyes. Sorry to say, this kept me from using anything to remove my eye makeup for years. I would sleep with it, and use dry tissues to wipe off the raccoon eyes the next morning. I do not recommend this. It gave me early wrinkles, which were later fixed by apple cider vinegar and coconut oil, and a lighter pigment around my eyes. Lesson learned!

Now I always remove my mascara at bedtime. You can use either olive oil or coconut oil or a combination of the two. Both are great at removing mascara and eye makeup, even the waterproof type. As an added benefit, they moisturize the undereye area and help remove or prevent wrinkles.

Exfoliate

Exfoliants are creams and scrubs that slough off dead skin cells, leaving your skin soft and glowing. Many commercial exfoliants contain chemicals (or the environmentally unsound microbeads) and can be quite expensive, so I definitely recommend that you make your own. Here are some wonderfully effective options:

Honey Mask Facial. Take a warm shower or hold your face over a bowl of steaming water to open pores. Rub warm honey on your face and let it sit for 20 to 30 minutes. Rinse with warm water and splash with cool water to close pores. Honey also works great as a gentle face wash that can be used every day.

Food Facial Mask. No need to drop a lot of money at the spa for great skin; just rub breakfast on your face instead! Use honey, plain yogurt, or whipped egg whites by themselves or in combination for a great toning facial mask, and watch your skin glow.

Sugar Scrub. Sugar is harmful for your body, but applied externally, it is a wonderful exfoliant and an effective way to tighten and smooth your skin. To make your own inexpensive sugar scrub, mix equal parts of white or brown sugar and olive or almond oil together. If you wish, add a few drops of essential oils to the mix. Then simply rub the mixture onto your skin and massage in for a couple of minutes. Rinse off with warm water. Your skin will be smooth and clear.

Baking Soda. This common household product is a natural microdermabrasion agent. It acts as a gentle agent that sloughs off dead skin cells and makes your skin glow. Wet your face with warm water. Sprinkle a little baking soda onto your hands and massage into your face for at least 3 minutes. Rinse with warm water and pat dry.

Tone

Although commercial toners don't ordinarily contain high levels of chemicals as other beauty products do, there are a couple of natural options that outperform conventional products by far and make you look a lot younger:

Diluted Organic Apple Cider Vinegar. Rubbing this vinegar on a freshly clean face makes a great toner. Make sure you dilute it with water, however. A teaspoon of vinegar per $\frac{1}{2}$ cup water is a good ratio. Add a few drops of essential oil to counter the smell (which will fade as soon as it dries). Apple cider vinegar tightens, brightens, and freshens your skin. Plus, it prevents dry skin and blemishes.

Witch Hazel. Here is another excellent toner and it can be used directly on the skin. Gentle and ideal for all skin types, witch hazel helps tighten and minimize pores and protects your skin from free-radical damage.

Moisturize

Each night before you go to bed, apply a moisturizer to your skin as the last step in this regimen, especially if you have dry skin. Remember too that oil cleansing functions as a moisturizer, so you may get to skip this step.

Commercial lotions can be loaded with harmful chemicals, many of which can be absorbed by the skin and stored in fat tissue. This is especially a concern for pregnant women, since these chemicals can be passed to a baby through the placenta. Swap out commercial lotions for natural options, and you'll avoid exposure to potential toxins.

The best natural lotions I have found so far are pure organic oils like argan, jojoba, olive, and coconut (or a mixture of these). These penetrate the skin well and help with wrinkles, dryness, and other skin problems.

SAVE FACE: THE GUT-SKIN CONNECTION

Your skin and digestive tract are linked, so if you want beautiful skin, you need a beautiful gut. The reason that many of us have stubborn skin problems such as acne or eczema has to do with tiny, unseen pathogenic (bad) bacteria in our guts. You can boost your gut health—and thus your skin—with the following:

- **Good-Quality Probiotics.** Probiotic supplements help replenish the good, skin-friendly bacteria in your gut. I always look for a high-quality spore-based probiotic. We also rotate probiotics as there is evidence that the gut can adapt to specific strains if they are taken continuously. We also focus on probiotic-rich foods and drinks like sauerkraut and beet kvass, which are a natural source of probiotics as well.

- **Fat-Soluble Vitamins.** Once I added fermented cod liver oil to my daily regimen years ago, my skin improved over time. I also noticed I got fewer stretch marks when I was taking this supplement during pregnancy and using natural products on my stomach.

- **Gelatin/Collagen.** I'm a big fan of gelatin and collagen powder for many reasons, but I credit these with speeding the healing of my skin from years of acne. I also often hear "You look way too young to have six kids," and I credit gelatin/collagen with these comments as well. Two great natural brands are Great Lakes and Vital Proteins.

- **L-Glutamine and Hydrochloride (HCL).** I also started taking L-glutamine, an amino acid that helps maintain the health of the digestive tract, for leaky gut and gut health, and it seemed to have a big impact on my skin as well. I still take L-glutamine daily on an empty stomach. I also still take betaine HCL to facilitate the repair of my intestines and support a healthy stomach.

MAKE YOUR OWN MAKEUP

It sounds difficult—making your own makeup. But once you get the hang of it, it's surprisingly easy, and you might have all of the ingredients in your kitchen already.

A good example is cocoa powder, which serves as a natural bronzer. Another is arrowroot, a thickener used in various food recipes. Using both of these, along with zinc oxide and cinnamon powder (another kitchen staple), you can create a natural power foundation in a shade very close to your skin color. Adding gold mica powder gives the foundation an even smoother texture and turns your skin radiant. See my Powdered Mineral Foundation recipe on page 191.

Try making your own natural liquid foundation. You can use my recipe, formulated with shea butter and argan oil, along with natural minerals and clays. It provides great coverage and looks beautiful on the skin. See page 194 for the full Natural Liquid Foundation formula.

MAKE A BASE MOISTURIZER

It's often a good idea to apply a moisturizer prior to putting on your foundation. There are actually two options for the base of this recipe: You can use a natural store-bought moisturizer. Or try my Homemade Base Moisturizer on page 192.

NATURAL BRONZING

I make a strong case for using a natural bronzer on your skin because commercial suntan lotion is under fire, even though it does protect us from the sun's ultraviolet light. A 2015 review in the medical journal *Hormones* called out these products as endocrine disruptors, meaning they interfere with the action of natural hormones in the body. This leads to a variety of problems, such as reproductive impairments and female and male cancers. Some of the endocrine-disrupting chemicals in suntan lotions include oxybenzone, benzophenones, octyl methoxycinnamate, camphors, and PABA (para-aminobenzoic acid), according to this article.

Not to worry, though. You can create a beautifully natural tan by making your own bronzer at home. Simply mix together cocoa powder, cinnamon, and arrowroot (optional) until you get a shade you like. For me, this was at least half cocoa powder, 30 to 40 percent cinnamon, and a little arrowroot, but experiment to match your skin tone. Store the mixture in a small glass jar or tin and brush it onto your skin for an instant bronze look. Bonus: it smells good! You can also mix this into lotion for a liquid version.

Once you make and apply these natural skin savers, expect to see a difference in just a week—sometimes overnight. The results are so immediate that you'll be hooked on these methods, and your favorite cosmetics counter may have to close up shop.

Chapter 8

your hair: keep it shiny, thick, and luxurious

Having been pregnant several times, I've enjoyed the wonderful thick hair that accompanies pregnancy, only to see it thin again after birth, thanks to hormonal changes. Because I love thick hair, I started searching for and testing ways to naturally promote hair growth.

CONSUME ENOUGH PROTEIN

Protein is essential for hair growth, so eating enough protein ensures that the body has the necessary building blocks for hair. Foods such as meats, fish, eggs, and especially bone broth are excellent for hair growth. Meat contains iron, another nutrient that helps hair grow. These foods also contain necessary fats that help promote healthy hormones and healthy hair.

GET THE VITAMINS

Some vitamins help promote hair growth, most notably vitamin C and biotin. The body needs vitamin C to produce collagen, a structural protein necessary for healthy hair and skin. Vitamin C also helps the body absorb iron. Because the body can't manufacture vitamin C, it is one vitamin that must be obtained from food or supplements. Foods such as broccoli, spinach, and citrus all contain vitamin C.

Biotin (a B vitamin) can also promote faster and stronger hair growth, and it is also good for the skin. Biotin is involved in the proper digestion of fats and sugars. Eggs, nuts, berries, fish, and some vegetables all supply biotin, although in small amounts, so supplementation is a good idea.

UP THE GELATIN

Gelatin is largely composed of the amino acids glycine and proline, which are found in the bones, fibrous tissues, and organs of animals—parts that Americans generally don't consume anymore. These amino acids are needed not only for proper skin, hair, and nail growth but also for optimal immune function and weight regulation. An easy way to consume gelatin is to blend about a teaspoon of the unflavored variety into a smoothie. The gelatin also helps make the smoothie even smoother!

BALANCE YOUR HORMONES FOR BETTER HAIR

Hormones are often a major cause of hair loss or poor hair growth, and unfortunately, there can be many causes of hormone imbalance. Of course, some steps can be taken to improve hair while working to balance hormones, and these are my top tips for regulating hormones naturally:

Eat quality fats. One of the best is coconut oil. Other quality sources of fats include avocados, animal fats, olive oil, grass-fed meats, pastured eggs, and raw dairy (for those who tolerate it). Quality seafood is also very important, because it is nature's best source of naturally occurring omega-3s.

Limit caffeine. I love coffee, but the truth is that too much caffeine can disrupt your hormone balance, especially if there are other hormone stressors involved, such as pregnancy, the presence of toxins, bad fats, or everyday stress.

Avoid harmful chemicals. Pesticides, plastics, household cleaners, and even mattresses can contain hormone-disrupting chemicals that mimic hormones in the body and keep the body from producing real hormones.

Prioritize sleep. I can't emphasize this one enough. Without adequate sleep, hormones will not be in balance. Period.

Supplement. Consider hormone-helping supplements such as maca, magnesium, vitamin D$_3$, omega-3 fats, and others your doctor may recommend.

TRY DRY SHAMPOO FOR HAIR HEALTH

Washing your hair too much (like every day) can strip it of natural oils that keep hair healthy looking. Here's where dry shampoos can help. Dry shampoos can make your hair look clean when it hasn't been washed for a while.

Dry shampoos are also great if you're switching to "no-poo" or homemade natural shampoo, which can leave your hair oily for the first week or so while your scalp adjusts to not having its natural oils stripped each day. I have naturally oily hair even when I don't strip the oils, so I am a huge fan of dry shampoo.

The basic idea of a dry shampoo is to put an oil-absorbing substance (such as arrowroot or cornstarch) on the oily parts of your hair to temporarily absorb the oil and leave your hair looking clean. This is also very helpful if you'll be styling hair and need it to hold. Dirty hair holds better than clean hair, but it doesn't have to *look* dirty.

Another option is a wet-dry shampoo. It uses the same concept, but puts the oil-absorbing substance in a quickly evaporating liquid like vodka or rubbing alcohol (or rum if you want to smell like a pirate).

Commercial dry shampoos can be pricey and contain harsh chemicals such as isobutane, butane, and propane—which is why I recommend making your own. You'll not only save money since homemade versions are about 95 percent cheaper, but you won't be putting explosive chemicals on your hair.

On my hair, I use a light powder (arrowroot) since I'm blonde, but for dark hair, cocoa powder mixed with arrowroot works better (plus, you get to smell like chocolate—win-win!). Arrowroot works for dark hair too.

NATURAL SHAMPOOS

The best ingredient for making your own shampoo is soap nuts. These are very inexpensive and work on all hair types. Find my recipes for natural shampoo in Chapter 19.

NATURAL COLOR ENHANCEMENT

You can enhance your hair color naturally by using certain herbs. I started out with sandy blonde hair, so I've used lightening herbs on most of my head, and I'm the blondest I've been since childhood (with some interesting red/brown streaks underneath).

My blonde/light recipes permanently lighten your hair since they naturally bleach it, but the red and dark hues will leave a temporary tint for a few weeks (depending on how often you wash it). The sun will help set all the hues.

Caveat: I haven't tried these recipes on dyed or chemically treated hair, so I don't know how it will react.

Herbs for Light Hair

I've tried several basic herbal variations, including:

- Strong chamomile tea (brewed with $1/2$ cup herbs per 2 cups water), which is cooled and then sprayed or poured on hair and left on for several hours. Sitting in the sun during this time enhances the lightening effect.

- Fresh squeezed lemon juice, sprayed and brushed through hair and left on for several hours (in the sun), also produces natural highlights.

- A chamomile tea rinse at the end of each shower (leave in your hair!) will produce smooth, silky hair and naturally lighter hair over time.

Herbs for Dark Brown Hair or Black Hair

If you have very light hair, it will be difficult to get really dark hues with just herbs, but with enough patience, it can be done. I've listed herbs that work, and you can use them in any combination. As always, test on a small section of hair before using. Henna hair colors will provide really dark results that last longer, but if you want to go dark gradually, here are some methods I've tried:

For very dark hair, place $1/4$ cup black walnut powder in a tea bag or cheesecloth bag and steep in 3 cups boiling water in a quart-size mason jar for at least 6 hours or overnight. Use as a rinse in the shower for hair and dry in the sun if possible. This will create very dark hair, especially if you have dry hair. It will also

HAIR CONDITIONER. Blend together avocado and coconut milk or cream in a blender and apply to dry hair. Leave on for up to 30 minutes, then rinse.

HAIR RINSE. Instantly clarify and remove oils from your hair by mixing 1 part white vinegar with 5 parts distilled water. Add 5 to 10 drops of your favorite essential oil for a fresh scent. I recommend lavender, lemon, orange, or peppermint. Pour this mixture over hair after shampooing or conditioning it. Depending on your hair type, you may also benefit from detoxing your hair with healing clays and using a natural shampoo.

OILY HAIR REPAIR. For oily hair, massage baking soda into your hair; shampoo as normal and rinse. This can be drying for some people and irritating to the scalp. If you want a gentler option, also try DIY dry shampoo for dark or light hair (see pages 203–204).

provide the darkest coverage for gray hair. Repeat daily or as needed to darken and maintain dark shade.

Use strong brewed black tea as a final rinse to darken any color hair. This is also nourishing for the hair and will provide a temporary darkening effect on most hair types. Repeat as necessary to get desired shade and sun-dry if possible.

With any of these herbal hair colors, make sure to test on a small part of your hair first, especially with henna- and color-treated hair as they have more lasting effects. Experiment with mixtures to get the right combination for your hair. Recipes for other hair-coloring methods are found in Chapter 19.

A FASTER WAY

If you want faster and more permanent results, you can use henna hair color. I've purchased it from both Mountain Rose Herbs and Morrocco Method. They are both excellent products, and the results are very dramatic. They have a lot of color variations with red hues (and darker ones), and the results last for several months (or longer if you wash your hair less often). They won't completely cover gray hair, but will darken it. Don't use on chemically treated hair. Test on a small section before using on your whole head.

VOLUMIZING SEA SALT SPRAY

Sea salt spray (also called beach waves spray) has gained popularity lately. Many of the sea salt sprays are also drying to the hair, since salt pulls moisture and natural oils out. This type of spray is easy to make yourself. It costs about one-fiftieth of the store-bought versions and adds great texture and volume to hair without the chemicals. If you make it yourself, you can also customize to your hair type to get the texture you want. See my Sea Salt Texturizing Hair Spray on page 206.

YOU CAN MAKE YOUR OWN NATURAL HAIR SPRAY

Hair spray is one of the worst offenders when it comes to chemicals in beauty products. It typically has aerosol, plastics, and more. Luckily, as with most beauty products, there is a simple, natural, and easy-to-make alternative that is also less expensive and healthier for hair. Surprisingly, it uses only a few ingredients, including white sugar. You can find my Hair Spray recipe on page 207.

HAIR GROWTH

Many men notice thinning or balding hair as they age. Women typically only get the pleasure of this experience after a pregnancy (so much fun—you just created an entire human being and now you get to lose your hair too!).

When experimenting with natural ways to encourage hair regrowth for myself after a pregnancy, I realized that one of my concoctions would be just as effective on men and that many guys might like some help to avoid hair loss.

Natural Oils to Encourage Hair Growth

There are a variety of natural oils that encourage hair growth quickly and easily. In my Natural Hair Growth Oil recipe (page 208), I use these:

Castor Oil. Used for detoxification in remedies like castor oil packs, I've applied this oil to thicken and lengthen my hair and eyelashes. It works for guys too. Castor oil not only helps avoid hair loss, but it can double or triple nor-

mal hair growth rates (my hair grew 1½ inches in a month using it twice a week).

Black Seed Oil. Black seed oil has many benefits, but it is especially wonderful for hair growth. It can help remedy some fungal infections that lead to hair loss and may also help prevent thinning hair. It can be used internally or topically; just test a small amount on the skin of your inner arm to make sure there is no sensitivity before using on the head or any large area of the body.

Rosemary Oil. Well known for its ability to stimulate hair growth, rosemary is often added to hair-growth treatments and shampoos. Adding a small amount creates a manly smell and increases the effectiveness of this recipe.

Lavender Essential Oil. Also useful for improving skin health and hair growth, lavender oil helps mellow out the scent of the black cumin seed and rosemary to create a refreshing but still manly scent.

Optional Olive Oil + Cayenne (2 tablespoons of olive oil infused with ½ teaspoon ground cayenne pepper). If you opt to use this, heat the oil slightly over a double burner and add the cayenne. Allow to infuse over low heat for 30 minutes and strain out the cayenne. Alternatively, you can leave the cayenne and oil in a glass jar in the sun for a few days to make a solar-infused oil and then strain as normal. Cayenne helps boost blood circulation and is a folk remedy for hair loss and sore muscles.

I find it amazing that you can do anything to your hair, from shampooing to conditioning to coloring, with items found mostly in your kitchen. Best of all, these products work better than their more expensive, store-bought counterparts. You'll love the results.

Chapter 9

your body: bathe your way to beauty

Nothing is more relaxing than a warm detoxification bath that draws toxins from your body. If you struggle with toxins or skin issues, recipes that employ salts, baking soda, apple cider vinegar, and other natural ingredients are a simple, easy, and inexpensive way to boost your health.

VINEGAR BATHS

There are many types of baths that can be used for detoxification and relaxation, but none benefits the skin as much as a vinegar bath. I'm not a fan of the smell of vinegar, but I'm a huge fan of vinegar baths because they leave my skin looking and feeling amazing.

The best vinegar to use is apple cider vinegar—for several reasons. First, it is a natural source of B vitamins, vitamin C, and trace minerals, making it nourishing to skin.

Second, apple cider vinegar is naturally acidic, so it helps balance the skin's pH, which should be slightly acidic. Also, many people with joint problems notice improvement from soaking in apple cider vinegar baths, and these beneficial acids and vitamins may be part of the reason.

Third, apple cider vinegar soothes skin problems. It can help naturally kill fungus and bacteria on the skin and offers relief for many with eczema and other skin conditions, including dandruff, dry skin, and pimples.

Finally, apple cider vinegar baths are often recommended for the treatment of urinary tract infections. Vinegar can help kill the yeast or fungus and create an environment in which it is difficult for infection to thrive. (For this reason, apple cider vinegar is also a potential remedy for warts and athlete's foot.)

Once or twice a week, I fill a tub with warm to hot water and add 1 to 2 cups of apple cider vinegar. I soak for 20 to 30 minutes, using a washcloth to clean my face and making sure to get my hair wet as well. After bathing, I rinse off in a cool shower, though some sources recommend letting the vinegar water dry on the skin. Experiment with both methods to see what works best for you.

AFTER BATHING: DETOX YOUR ARMPITS—AND YOUR BODY

Take your detoxification one step further with an "armpit detox." It can help pull chemicals and toxins left by commercial deodorants and antiperspirants from the skin and tissue of your armpits.

You see, conventional deodorants and antiperspirants contain a variety of chemicals and additives. Unnatural substances like these block the body's natural ability to sweat—which is important to detoxification.

In fact, the list of chemicals in some deodorants is scary and includes aluminum (implicated in cancer and Alzheimer's disease), phthalates, propylene glycol (which is essentially antifreeze), formaldehyde (a known carcinogen), parabens, and antibacterial chemicals.

The detox involves mixing 1 tablespoon bentonite clay, 1 teaspoon apple cider vinegar, and 1 to 2 teaspoons water. Apply this mixture to your armpits and let it stay there for 15 to 20 minutes. Then wash it off.

Several friends and I tried this detox, and here's what we found:

- We all noticed less odor, even without wearing any deodorant afterward.

- All but one person said she noticed less sweat.

- Everyone said they would recommend it to a friend.

Of course, our "scientific" experiment was informal and somewhat less than scientific, but for my friends and me, the results seemed promising.

Because antiperspirant and deodorant products are some of the worst offenders when it comes to beauty products, you might want to consider making your own and using them. Homemade versions will not infiltrate your body with chemicals and will let you detox naturally.

A simple homemade deodorant can be whipped with baking soda and coconut oil. Baking soda by itself is actually an incredibly effective natural deodorant, although it can be messy if you're wearing a dark color. Mixing baking soda with an equal part of coconut oil is a cleaner option. Because coconut oil has antibacterial and antifungal properties, it is effective at preventing odor. See Chapter 19 for several other natural deodorant formulas.

You can also buy natural alternatives, but look out for any containing aluminum of any kind, and check yours in the EWG Skin Deep Database before buying.

DRY BRUSHING FOR BEAUTIFUL SKIN AND GLORIOUS HEALTH

You probably brush your hair and your teeth (hopefully with natural toothpaste, but if not, see Chapter 10), but do you brush your skin? And why would you?

Dry brushing is exactly what it sounds like: brushing your skin in a particular pattern with a dry brush, usually before showering. In dry brushing, the skin is typically brushed toward your heart, starting at your feet and hands and brushing toward your chest.

I've been dry brushing my skin for years, mostly because it feels great and makes my skin softer, but there are other benefits as well.

Lymphatic Support

The lymphatic system is a major part of the body's immune system. It is made up of organs and lymph nodes, ducts, and vessels that transport lymph throughout the body. Many of these lymph vessels run just below the skin, and proponents of dry brushing claim that brushing the skin regularly stimulates normal lymph flow and helps the body detoxify itself naturally.

Exfoliation

You'll notice this benefit the first time you dry-brush. Running a firm, natural-bristled brush over your skin helps loosen and remove dead skin cells, naturally exfoliating skin. I noticed much softer skin in the first few days and weeks after I started dry brushing, and my skin has stayed soft. Dry brushing is one of the simplest and most natural ways to exfoliate skin. I love this benefit of skin brushing and how soft my skin feels when I do this regularly.

An added benefit of exfoliating the skin in this manner is that it clears oil, dirt, and residue from the pores. I use a specialized smaller gentler dry brush for my face. After brushing, my facial skin is softer, and my pores are much less noticeable.

Minimize Cellulite

Though the evidence is anecdotal, I've read many accounts of people who claim that regular dry brushing greatly helped their cellulite. There isn't much research to back the cellulite claims, but dry brushing feels great and makes skin softer, so there isn't really any downside to trying it.

Boost Energy Naturally

I can't explain why, but dry brushing always gives me a natural energy boost. For this reason, I wouldn't recommend dry brushing at night, but it is great in the morning. One theory is that because it increases circulation, it also increases energy. Either way, dry brushing is part of my morning routine.

How to Select a Dry Brush

I use a firm, natural-bristle brush with a handle, which allows me to reach my entire back and easily brush the bottoms of my feet and the backs of my legs.

Steps for Dry Brushing

1. Starting at your feet, brush the bottoms and up your legs in long, smooth strokes. Brush each section of skin ten times. For lymph flow, brush toward your heart/chest area where the

lymph system drains. As a good rule of thumb, always brush toward the center of the body.

2. Repeat the same process with your arms, starting with the palms of your hands and brushing up your arm toward the heart. Again, brush each section of skin ten times.

3. On your stomach and armpits, brush in a circular clockwise motion.

4. Repeat the process on your abdomen and back and on your face with a smaller, more delicate brush.

Note: Don't brush too hard! A soft and smooth stroke often works best. My skin is slightly pink after brushing, but it should never be red or sting. If it hurts at all, apply less pressure. Replace your brush every 6 to 12 months because the bristles will eventually wear out. I also recommend washing the brush every few weeks to remove dead skin cells.

A bath routine using a natural brush, followed by an armpit detox and dry brushing, is a simple and effective way to wash away impurities and stress. Use this protocol, and you'll be easily on your way to a less toxic life.

Chapter 10

your teeth and gums: keep a beautiful smile for life

Are you preparing for a big night on the town? A job interview? Or do you just want to look your best? Although gorgeous clothes may accent your value, and flawless makeup and a great hairstyle may glam you up, the most important component in good looks can't be found at the spa, salon, or shopping mall. That can be found only in an attractive smile, which will beautify your appearance and boost your self-esteem and also enhance other people's impression of you. Even more important is your gum health. Many people may have the early signs of gum disease and not even realize it. Symptoms like persistent bad breath, swollen gums, gums that bleed when flossing, sensitive teeth, or painful spots on the gums when chewing can all be early signs of gum disease.

According to David Kennedy, DDS, and past president of the International Association for Oral Medicine and Toxicology, more than 90 percent of adults over age thirty have some stage of active gum disease, and more alarming, 65 percent of fifteen-year-olds already have active gum disease.

It is well established that gum disease can be devastating to the mouth and is the leading cause of adult tooth loss and other oral problems. What is less well known is that gum disease can also have negative impact on other parts of the body. The mouth is not an isolated ecosystem but an integral part of the immune system. It is intimately connected to many other parts of the body, and a bacterial imbalance or gum disease in the mouth can create immune problems and inflammation in other parts of the body as well.

Luckily, regular at-home dental care, including oil pulling and other natural remedies, can help prevent gum disease, and possibly reverse it.

OIL PULLING: A PREVENTIVE PAYOFF

An age-old remedy rooted in Ayurvedic medicine, oil pulling uses natural substances to clean and detoxify teeth and gums. The practice of oil pulling (also called *gundusha*) started in India thousands of years ago and, from my research, was first introduced to the United States in the early 1990s by a medical doctor named Dr. F. Karach, who used it with success in his medical practice.

Oil pulling has the added effect of whitening teeth naturally. Also, evidence shows that it may be beneficial for gum health and that certain oils may help fight harmful bacteria in the mouth.

Here's how it works: Oil pulling is the act of swishing oil (usually sesame, sunflower, or coconut) in your mouth for up to twenty minutes. The oil is able to cut through plaque and remove toxins without disturbing the teeth or gums. Do this daily or 1 to 2 times a week.

If your goal is whitening the teeth, I've found coconut oil to be most effective. Coconut oil is also slightly more effective at removing certain bacteria from the mouth, including *Streptococcus mutans,* which is known for causing dental cavities.

Sesame oil is recommended by most sources (though this is partially because it was one of the more widely available oils when the practice first started years ago). It is also the most widely studied and considered safe for those who are not allergic to sesame seeds.

Olive oil is sometimes used, though some sources claim that it is too harsh for the teeth.

The main thing is to avoid using any oils high in omega-6 or chemically created oils like vegetable oil, canola oil, soybean oil, corn oil, and others.

Benefits of Oil Pulling

Oil pulling seems to be a practice with a plethora of anecdotal support but a lack of extensive scientific studies. Most sources agree that oil pulling is safe but debate how effective it is. Though more research is needed to determine any scientific backing to oil pulling, I've noticed the benefits personally and many of my readers swear by its effectiveness as well.

In fact, in my original research, I found hundreds of testimonials online from people who experienced benefits from oil pulling, including help with skin conditions, arthritis, asthma, headaches, hormone imbalances, infections, liver problems, and more.

Although I've used oil pulling for a few years, my only personal experience is with increased oral health (no plaque) and less sensitive (and whiter) teeth. I've heard several experts explain how bacteria and infection can enter the blood through the mouth, so it makes sense that addressing these infections could have an impact in other parts of the body.

Oil pulling may also remineralize the teeth; however, more research is needed. I did use oil pulling as part of a protocol to remineralize my teeth, but I suspect that the benefit may have stemmed from the ability of certain oils to combat the bacteria that causes tooth decay rather than actual mineral support for the tooth.

Coconut and sesame oils, for example, are not excellent sources of the minerals that teeth need, so using them in the mouth wouldn't be a very effective way to provide minerals for the teeth. Because the mouth is constantly protecting and replenishing the minerals in teeth and enamel through saliva, it seems much more important to make sure the body is getting enough minerals internally so that they are available in saliva.

What about bad breath? Yes, oil pulling does improve breath. In fact, this is one benefit all sources seem to agree on: Oil has the ability to help wipe out harmful bacteria in the mouth.

At the very least, I think that oil pulling can be beneficial and has no downside as long as a quality oil (that is high enough quality to eat) is used and it is done correctly. Oil pulling is a very inexpensive therapy that could potentially have great benefit on oral health, so there's no downside in trying it.

Steps for Oil Pulling

1. Put 1 to 2 teaspoons oil into your mouth. I also add a few drops of peppermint, cinnamon, or clove essential oil into the mix.

2. Swish the oil for 20 minutes. This is long enough to break through plaque and bacteria but not long enough that the body starts reabsorbing the toxins and bacteria. The oil gets thicker and milkier as it mixes with your saliva; it should be creamy white when spit out. Because it doubles in volume while you're swishing, it can be difficult at first to do it for a full 20 minutes. Don't worry, though. Just do only 5 or 10 minutes at first, and gradually build up to 20 minutes.

3. Spit the oil into a trash can, not into the sink. The oil may thicken and clog pipes (especially if you have a septic system like mine). Do not swallow the oil because it will be full of bacteria, toxins, and pus that you'll want to expel from your mouth.

4. Rinse your mouth well with warm water. In my opinion, warm water seems to clean the mouth better. Swish a few times to remove any remaining oil. Some sources recommend swishing with warm salt water.

5. Brush well.

Who Can Do Oil Pulling?

Children. Several practitioners I've asked said that oil pulling is safe for kids once they are old enough not to swallow the oil.

Pregnant Women. I've done oil pulling during pregnancy, but I was also doing it regularly before I got pregnant. I asked a midwife and she said that it is generally considered safe for pregnant women, especially after the first trimester. Oral health is especially important during pregnancy, so I've always considered it an extra benefit to my usual brushing and mouthwash routine. (Purely anecdotal: I haven't had a cavity since I started oil pulling and my oral health routine.) As with anything, check with a doctor or midwife before doing oil pulling, especially if pregnant.

Nursing. During this period, oil pulling is generally considered safe, but check with a dentist or doctor to be on the safe side.

Dental Issues. I have several non-amalgam fillings in my mouth and got the okay from my dentist and doctor to do oil pulling. Check with your doctor or dentist to be sure, especially if you have any metal fillings, crowns, or dental problems.

Note: Some people have reportedly noticed a detox reaction for the first few days after oil pulling, with symptoms that include mild congestion, headache, mucous drainage, or other effects. I personally have not experienced any of these effects but have read cases of others who did.

WHITEN YOUR TEETH NATURALLY

It sounds counterintuitive, but activated charcoal can do wonders for whitening teeth. I've also found it is great for gums and for overall oral health. This isn't a remedy that should be used daily because charcoal can be slightly abrasive. I use this once a week to keep teeth white.

Purchase a bottle of supplements of activated charcoal. Break open a few capsules onto a dish. Dip your toothbrush in the charcoal powder and brush away. Rinse. This natural method is healthier than applying expensive, chemical-laden whiteners to your teeth.

Following a regular routine of natural dental care is an excellent form of detoxification. It helps prevent nasty bacteria and other toxins from entering your bloodstream and doing systematic damage. Plus, you're not ingesting chemicals that may be found in commercial dental products. It's definitely a win-win for everyone in your family.

STEP 3: *clean up without chemicals*

Now we're going to take a deep dive into the chemicals and toxins found in and around your home, particularly in the products you normally use to keep it clean. You'll discover how to limit your exposure to harsh chemicals in everyday products that you probably took for granted. I'll unveil ways to limit your exposure, make your own natural cleaning supplies, and help you take further control of your health. Welcome to Step 3!

Chapter 11

use natural household products

Every day our bodies are bombarded with hundreds of chemicals from paint, furniture, electrical goods, and even carpets. Many have been linked to headaches, allergies, asthma, and more serious problems. It's time to turn your home into a healthful haven. And it doesn't have to be a lot of work. Little changes can have a huge impact on the way you feel. We spend an average of 90 percent of our lives indoors, so it pays to get things right.

As the number of household cleaning products has jumped, so have the unsafe chemical combinations in those products. Most cleaning products you buy in the store have long ingredient lists of harsh chemicals: bleach, ammonia, and acids, to name a few. Store-bought cleaners can give off fumes that can irritate your eyes, skin, and lungs. Children and pets are particularly vulnerable. Some products also contain unnecessary antibacterial agents that can promote the growth of antibacterial-resistant organisms. But the good news is that you can replace these synthetic products with natural nontoxic versions you can make at home. They work just as well, if not better, and are less expensive.

BAKING SODA

Baking soda, or sodium bicarbonate, is a highly alkaline salt. It has a slightly bitter, salty taste and is often used in baking because of its ability to react with an acid to create carbon dioxide gas, which creates "fluffiness" in the finished recipe.

There are dozens of household uses for baking soda. Following are just a few.

Natural Oven Cleaning

Baking soda makes a great oven cleaner. Simply spray the whole oven with water so that it is damp, and sprinkle on a $1/4$-inch layer of baking soda on the bottom of the oven. Mist it with a water bottle so that none of the baking soda layer is dry.

Leave the baking soda in place for a few hours (with the oven off). Then wipe off the paste with a cloth. Watch how all the grime comes off with it. Stubborn grime may take a few more applications.

Scouring Powder

Baking soda, borax, and salt make an effective and natural scouring powder that takes even the toughest stains off tubs and floors. Simply mix equal parts—and scrub away.

Tough Tile and Grout Cleaning

When we moved into our first real house, the 1960s tile needed some serious love, and the grout was stained and gross. These natural tile and grout cleaners did the trick:

Light Cleaning of Water Spots or Dirt. Get a damp sponge, dip it in a bowl of regular baking soda, and wipe down tub or tiles. Rinse with warm water.

Tough Stains or Set-In Dirt. Use a damp sponge soaked in full-strength white vinegar to wipe down entire surface. Immediately scour with baking soda and a brush or sponge.

Really Tough Stains and Spots. Mix $1/2$ cup baking soda with 2 tablespoons washing soda and 2 tablespoons borax. Add 3 tablespoons liquid castile soap and stir (if you don't have

8 MORE AMAZING USES FOR BAKING SODA

- Scrub or soak your hair brushes in a mixture of baking soda and warm water to degrease and clean them.

- Use the oven-cleaning method described at left to remove goop and grease from pans.

- Keep baking soda next to your stove to extinguish grease fires.

- Dab a little baking soda mixed with water on a bug bite or itch to ease the itch.

- Pour some baking soda in the garbage disposal with the rind of a fresh lemon and run the disposal to freshen.

- Soak toothbrushes in 1 tablespoon baking soda dissolved in 1 cup water for 2 to 4 hours and "rinse" with hydrogen peroxide to kill germs. I especially like to do this after someone has been ill.

- Use baking soda in place of rock salt on icy sidewalks.

- Use baking soda as a natural antacid. Stir $1/4$ teaspoon baking soda in an 8-ounce glass of water to neutralize heartburn or indigestion.

liquid castile soap, you can use liquid dish soap). Prewipe with full-strength white vinegar, and scrub with the baking-soda mixture. For tubs, wipe with white vinegar, sprinkle with the mixture, and let sit for 15 minutes. Scrub with heavy-duty brush and rinse.

Moldy Grout Stains. For mold on grout, make a mixture of 1 part 3% hydrogen peroxide and 1 part water in a spray bottle. Spray on grout until saturated. Wait 45 minutes and wipe down with sponge. Rinse well.

WHITE VINEGAR

Several years ago, after I switched to all-natural cleaning products, I found that one of the products I use the most when cleaning is distilled white vinegar (it is also available in organic versions). I know, I know, you don't want your house to smell like pickles, but don't worry, the smell fades when it dries and can be easily masked with a few drops of essential oil. Vinegar is an all-around effective cleaner.

Window Cleaner

Vinegar is by far more effective than other conventional glass cleaners at cleaning windows and mirrors and will yield a spot-free shine. I mix 1 part vinegar to 3 parts water and add a few drops of my favorite essential oil (lemongrass).

Mold Remover

One part borax mixed with 4 parts white vinegar in a spray bottle does wonders for mold. Just spray it on, wait about an hour, and wipe up. The mold sponges right off.

Hardwood Floors

Our last house had hardwood floors throughout, and this meant a lot of mopping for me. I found that $1/3$ to $2/3$ cup white vinegar mixed in 1 gallon warm water cleans hardwoods very quickly and easily.

Toilet Cleaning

Pour a few shakes of baking soda in the toilet bowl and add 1 cup vinegar. This combo will create a bubbly reaction that, when scrubbed, leaves the toilet shining.

Cleaning Cabinets

If you have food spots, oil buildup, or stains on your cabinets, mix 1 part vinegar with 3 parts water, and scrub with a rag or sponge. The vinegar will cut any grease, leaving the cabinets clean and shiny.

All-Purpose Cleaning

For everything else, I have two bottles of home-made spray cleaner in the kitchen and all bathrooms. One of these consists of $1/2$ cup white vinegar, 2 cups water, and 10 to 20 drops essential oil (optional). This does wonders on countertops, high-chair trays, baseboards, walls, appliances, floors, and everywhere else where messes can be dumped, spilled, or tracked.

Clothing Stains

Pour undiluted vinegar onto the stain and wash as normal. This method works effectively for wine, tomato sauce, or other spills on carpet. Immediately pour vinegar on the area, wait a few minutes, and wipe up with a damp cloth.

NATURAL STAIN REMOVER GUIDE

INK OR PAINT STAINS. Soak in rubbing alcohol for 30 minutes or (ink only) spray with Hair Spray (page 207), then wash out.

TEA OR COFFEE STAINS. Immediately pour boiling water over the stain until it is gone, or if it has already set, scrub with a paste of borax and water and wash immediately.

GRASS STAINS. Scrub with liquid dish soap, or treat with equal parts 3% hydrogen peroxide and water.

MUD STAINS. Let dry and brush off what you can, then scrub with a borax/water paste and wash immediately.

TOMATO-BASED STAINS. Apply white vinegar directly on the stain, then wash immediately.

DINGY WHITES OR UNDERARM DEODORANT STAINS. Presoak the stain directly in a mix of equal parts hydrogen peroxide and water for 30 minutes. Then add 1 cup hydrogen peroxide to the wash water. For really tough yellow stains, make a paste of equal parts 3% hydrogen peroxide and baking soda. Rub the paste into the stain, let sit for 5 minutes, then launder.

OTHER FOOD STAINS. Treat with a mix of equal parts hydrogen peroxide and water, and soak for at least 10 minutes.

GREASE AND OIL STAINS. Sprinkle the stain with baking soda to absorb any oil or grease, then brush off. Soak in undiluted white vinegar for 15 minutes, rinse, and scrub with liquid dish soap before washing

VOMIT, URINE, POOP, BLOOD, EGG, GELATIN, GLUE, OR OTHER PROTEIN-BASED STAINS. Do *not* wash in warm water—this will set in the smell. Soak in cool water for half an hour, then wash with an added mixture of ½ cup hydrogen peroxide and ½ cup baking soda in the washing machine.

REMOVE STAINS NATURALLY

If your household is anything like mine, laundry stains are a daily fact of life. Unfortunately, conventional laundry stain treatment solutions and removers are some of the most toxic cleaning products available. They contain harsh detergents, solvents, chemicals like sulfates and parabens, and a host of artificial colors and scents. So I don't recommend that you use them.

Borrowing some wisdom from my grandma's era and my professional stain creation experts (aka my children), I compiled a helpful list of effective stain treatments for various types of stains. I keep this list handy for reference when I'm doing laundry. Tip: Always treat stains from the back, rather than the front, to avoid rubbing the stain in more.

When used correctly, these methods are highly effective (and you won't have to keep the poison control number on hand!).

WASHING SODA

Washing soda (soda ash) is a natural cleaner and booster that can be used on its own or in various DIY recipes for natural cleaning. It is available in many grocery stores and online.

Chemically, washing soda is a highly alkaline substance with a unique chemical composition that makes it excellent for household uses like degreasing, brightening, and cleaning tough messes.

It scores an exceptional safety rating from the Environmental Working Group; the only warning is to use it safely, as you would any highly alkaline substance (e.g., not undiluted on skin, not consumed internally, and so forth).

Is Baking Soda the Same as Washing Soda?

In short . . . no!

Washing soda (sodium carbonate) is chemically much different and should be used in washing, cleaning, and household uses but never in food or baking.

The reason that washing soda is not used in baking and cooking is that it is stronger. It often reacts too strongly with the acid in the recipe, changing the taste or texture dramatically. This chemical difference, however, makes washing soda excellent for stain treating, homemade laundry detergent, and all-purpose cleaner. In fact, washing soda has dozens of household uses.

Laundry Booster

This is the original purpose of washing soda—for laundry. Add about $1/2$ cup to a load of laundry, especially whites, to clean, brighten, and deodorize.

Homemade Laundry Soap

Speaking of laundry (which we pretty much always are as moms, aren't we?), washing soda is one of the mainstays in my Fresh Lemon-Powdered Laundry Detergent (page 224) and Unscented Liquid Laundry Detergent (page 225) recipes, which I've been using for years. It's much more budget-friendly and natural than many commercial brands.

Grease Stains and Tough Stains

Washing powder's high alkaline properties make this simple white powder a dynamo at removing grease and other tough stains, especially when treated early. I sprinkle some directly on grease stains on clothes right before washing to pull out the stain. Baking soda is another option.

Note: Don't do this ahead of time and leave on the clothes too long—washing powder's alkaline pH can "eat" through fabrics.

All-Purpose Cleaner

Washing soda is also a core ingredient in my homemade Citrus-Fresh All-Purpose Cleaner (page 223), which naturally cleans almost anything.

Carpet Stains

We finally removed the very old, nasty carpet in our living room, but until then, I cleaned that thing more than I'd like to admit. I would sprinkle on some washing soda, let it absorb for 5 to 10 minutes, and vacuum it up. Please note that this worked on my white (or formerly white) carpet. Check with the manufacturer on your carpet or ask an expert prior to using any really strong substance like this on yours.

Turbo-Charged Presoak

Got some really nasty clothes or bad stains? Use washing soda as a presoak. Fill and start your laundry load as usual, but before starting, add 1 cup washing soda and let your laundry soak about 20 minutes.

Grill Cleaner

Its grease-busting power makes washing soda wonderful at cleaning outdoor grills. Ours gets burned into a scummy mess after only a month or two. To renew the shine, we remove the grills and soak them in a strong mixture of washing soda and water. Grease and burned-on food comes right off.

Blind Cleaner

Want a fast way to clean all the vinyl blinds in your house? Fill your bathtub with warm water. Add 1 cup washing soda. Remove all the blinds and soak for 30 minutes. Spray or wipe down with the cleaner and rehang. (From my experience, make a note of where they all go before doing this!)

Alternatively, dissolve ¼ cup washing soda in 2 quarts warm water and use to wipe down blinds while they are still hanging.

Pots and Pans Cleaner

Have stainless-steel pots or pans with stuck-on grease or burned-on stains? Let washing soda work its magic. Sprinkle on some washing soda; spray water with a fine-mist sprayer until a paste forms and let it sit for 20-plus minutes and scrub off.

Note: Do not do this with aluminum pans as it may leach out the aluminum.

Oven Cleaner

Just as with pots and pans, washing soda can remove burned-on and stuck-on food from the bottom of the oven. Use the oven-cleaning method described on page 76. Avoid getting washing soda paste on the actual heating element (the washing soda can wear down the heating element), and wash all residue out thoroughly with a wet cloth before using the oven.

Hard-Water Stains

As a natural water softener, washing soda also helps remove hard-water stains on sinks, appliances, faucets, or anywhere else they are. Just make a paste and scrub until the spots are gone.

Drain Cleaner

Once a week or so, I dump ½ cup washing soda down my kitchen sink drain to keep it unclogged and smelling fresh. If I have one, I'll also throw in a lemon rind and use the disposal to chop it up.

Range Hood Degreasing

A little washing soda sprinkled on a cloth or sponge takes off any grease stuck inside the range hood.

Trash Can Freshener

I keep my trash cans fresh by sprinkling a little washing soda in them every couple of weeks.

HYDROGEN PEROXIDE

One of the most versatile—and natural—cleaning solutions for the home is hydrogen peroxide, which can be used in a multitude of ways.

Make Toilet Bowls Sparkle

Remove dingy circles from your toilet bowls by pouring ½ cup hydrogen peroxide into the bowl. Let it stay there for 30 minutes, then easily scrub them away.

Get Whiter Whites

The whiter my white clothes, the better I like them. Hydrogen peroxide is my best friend here. Fill your sink three-quarters full of water and mix in ½ cup hydrogen peroxide. Add your whites, and let them soak for 10 minutes. Lightly scrub the clothes, then wash them with cold water.

Banish Bacteria from Your Refrigerator

To prevent bacteria buildup in your refrigerator, mix 5 tablespoons hydrogen peroxide with 1 gallon water. Wipe down the interior of your refrigerator to get rid of bacteria.

Shine Your Pots and Pans

Who hasn't experienced caked-on food in your pots and pans? To clean it off, mix 3 tablespoons hydrogen peroxide with 1 tablespoon baking soda to form a paste. Rub the paste onto your pots and pans. Leave it for 10 minutes or longer. Take a stainless-steel sponge and scrub—and the grime comes off like a charm.

Clean Your Sponges

Kitchen sponges we use over and over again can become breeding grounds for germs and bacteria because they are always moist. Prevent bacterial growth by soaking sponges in hydrogen peroxide after every use. Then wash them in your dishwasher as an extra precaution.

Remove Grout and Tile Stains

If your bathroom grout and tiles accumulate dirt and stains, you can remove them with hydrogen peroxide. Simply spray it, undiluted, onto the grout and tiles. Leave it there for 15 minutes, and then scrub off the stains.

Disinfect Countertops and Sinks

Hydrogen peroxide is masterful at removing soap residue and food stains from sinks. Combine 5 tablespoons hydrogen peroxide, 2 tablespoons baking soda, and ½ gallon water. Apply the mixture to a scouring sponge, and scrub the grime away easily.

Soak Vegetables

To remove soil and harmful chemicals from your vegetables, soak them in a solution of ¼ cup hydrogen peroxide and 1 gallon water. Soak your produce for about 20 minutes, and thoroughly rinse afterward.

LIQUID CASTILE SOAP

Named for the Castile region of Spain where soap was made from olive oil, liquid castile soap is very versatile and can replace many, if not all, of your commercially prepared, chemical-laden detergent cleaners. Most castile soap today is actually a mixture of olive oil, coconut oil, castor oil, or any other commonly used vegetable oil. Available as either a hard bar soap or a liquid soap, castile soap comes in several good brands. Dr. Bronner's is the most well known.

Hard soap bars are a result of mixing oils/fats and sodium hydroxide (lye). Liquid soaps are a result of mixing oils/fats and potassium hydroxide (caustic potash). Many people are concerned about using these caustic compounds and wonder how something can be "natural" when it contains them.

The beautiful thing about chemistry is that you can combine two substances to create a chemical reaction that yields an entirely new substance. Take salt, for example. Naturally occurring sea salt is a chemical compound consisting primarily of sodium and chloride. In its pure form, sodium is a metal that reacts violently when exposed to water, and chlorine is a poisonous green gas that has been used in chemical warfare. But together they are salt, a naturally occurring resource valuable and necessary for life.

The point here is that soap, if made properly, is a useful cleaning tool that is safe and gentle for use on your skin and for cleaning in your home. You are no more rubbing a caustic chemical on your skin than you are trying to clean your dishes with olive oil.

Here's a look at the many ways you can use liquid castile soap for home cleaning:

Mopping. Mix 2 tablespoons liquid castile soap and 1 gallon hot water in a bucket to mop your floor.

Hand-Washing Dishes. Add a squirt of liquid castile soap to hot running water when you are filling the sink to wash dishes. This won't bubble and suds up like a detergent would, but the soap is still in there doing its job. For tough, stuck-on food, allow dishes to soak for a little while before you scrub them.

Mirrors and Windows. Although it isn't necessary to use soap for regular mirror cleaning in your home, if you are switching from a commercial cleaner, you may need to add a few drops of liquid castile soap to your homemade window cleaner to remove the residue left by the commercial cleaner. Also, if you will be cleaning your exterior windows, the added castile soap will help clean away the grime and dirt they are exposed to all year long.

Bug Spray for Plants. Keep bugs away from your plants by spraying them with a mixture of 1 tablespoon liquid castile soap and 1 quart water. For an ant spray, increase the soap to ¼ cup and spray in problem areas. Just don't use this higher concentration on your plants because it will burn them.

BORAX

There's some debate surrounding borax and whether it's safe to use. Borax, of the mule team variety, is sodium tetraborate or sodium borate (to get official for a second); it is *not* boric acid (hydrogen borate), which is a common misconception on the interwebs apparently. Sodium tetraborate (hereafter referred to as borax) is a salt of boric acid, but it does not have the same chemical composition as boric acid. If you've read an article claiming borax is dangerous or that says borax and boric acid are the same thing, I would not consider that article credible.

Borax Versus Boric Acid

While both are used as natural pesticides, which is probably the reason for the misconception, boric acid carries a risk for toxicity at a much lower dose than borax does if ingested. To be clear, neither one should be ingested.

Borax is used in the process of making boric acid, but there is a tremendous chemical difference between the two. While borax is a naturally occurring mineral, that doesn't make it inert or wholly safe. Arsenic is a naturally occurring metalloid, but it isn't safe for human use. *Naturally occurring* doesn't always mean "safe."

Borax is extremely alkaline, which makes it irritating when used undiluted. So it makes sense to not use any form—borax, sodium borate, or boric acid—as an eye wash, skin scrub, or drink, but it doesn't answer the question about the safety of occasional indirect contact (as when used for cleaning products).

Here's a summary of what I learned when conducting my own research:

- Actual warnings for borax use relate to avoiding eye contact, undiluted skin contact, and ingestion.

- Borax is currently banned for food use by the FDA and in Europe. Though it has a history of use in food products, it is now listed as a substance of high concern and studies have shown that when ingested it can lead to short-term problems like digestive upset and long-term effects like developmental and reproductive delays.

- I was unable to find any studies that proved borax to be a danger in natural cleaning products in diluted amounts.

- The Skin Deep Cosmetics Database classifies borax as a moderate hazard, but most of the studies and listings are related to borax use in food.

The Bottom Line: Is Borax Safe?

Most products I use borax in (like my all-purpose cleaner and laundry detergents) aren't coming in direct, undiluted contact with my skin, I'm not ingesting them, and I'm not getting them in or near my eyes, so most of the concerns and warnings with borax do not apply. If you aren't comfortable using borax, you can make natural cleaning products without it, but be sure to wear gloves when handling borax.

I still consider borax safe for use in natural cleaning, but I encourage you to do your own research and make sure you are using it in a safe capacity. I use a natural borax powder from Mountain Rose Herbs, so it is free of any added surfactants or detergents, but the Mule

Team brand is also considered a pure/natural form of borax.

STORING YOUR NATURAL CLEANERS

I prefer to use glass bottles over plastic bottles to store my natural cleaners. They last longer, and if I use any of the citrus essential oils in my cleaning products, they will eventually break down the plastic. So I keep plenty of glass spray bottles on hand for exactly this purpose. You can even create your own glass spray bottle by using an empty apple cider vinegar bottle fitted with a spray-bottle top.

SWITCH TO A PAPER-FREE KITCHEN

Switching to a paper-free kitchen and setting up a good system for using cloth is a great way to save money and be more environmentally friendly. I have cloth napkins, microfiber cloths, and huck towels in easily accessible places around the kitchen so that even the kids can use them. We keep cloth napkins by the table in a cabinet and huck towels and microfiber cloths in a drawer by the sink. Used towels are kept in a basket in the pantry until I am ready to run a load of laundry.

With our family size, I've found it helpful to keep the following on hand:

- 2 dozen or more huck towels

- 1 dozen microfiber cloths

- 3 to 4 dozen cloth napkins

- Other assorted cloths for cleaning and picking up spills, including cut-up old shirts, old cloth diapers/inserts, or old socks (for younger kids to use in cleaning and polishing)

I think the idea of removing paper products from the kitchen is much more daunting than the actuality. I have many friends who use cloth diapers but who still resist the idea of using cloth instead of paper towels and napkins in the kitchen (kitchen messes are less gross than poopy diapers in my opinion—at least most of the time!).

If you've never considered the idea of using cloth in the kitchen before, I'd encourage you to give it a try. Not only does it save money and reduce waste, but I actually find that it isn't much extra work at all (and we cook three times a day).

What Kind of Cloth?

I think the two biggest factors that make using cloth in the kitchen easy for us are picking the right kind of cloth and having enough of them on hand. To go paper-free in the kitchen, you have to find suitable replacements for paper napkins, paper towels, and other disposable products like cleaning wipes. I've found that there isn't necessarily a single solution that replaces all of these, but that there are very effective replacements for each category.

- Instead of paper napkins, use cloth napkins or microfiber cloths.

- Instead of paper towels, use huck towels or microfiber cloths.

- Instead of regular dish towels, use huck towels.

All paper products can be replaced by huck towels or microfiber cloths if you don't mind how they look as napkins. I've found that both of these are more absorbent than paper towels or paper napkins and surprisingly easy to use.

I like microfiber cloths because they are naturally antibacterial and seem to last forever (I've had mine over a year), but even the big economy packs in the auto section at stores like Sam's and Costco work great for kitchen messes.

If you haven't heard of huck towels before, I can't recommend them enough. We received a few from a friend for our wedding, and though I searched for years in home stores, I couldn't find them. Then I noticed them in an odd place: the hospital. Turns out, these are the type of towels they use in the hospital for absorbing blood and other fluids during and after surgery. You can order huck towels online, and they work wonderfully as regular kitchen towels and in place of paper towels.

The Laundry Aspect

My biggest hesitation in switching to cloth was the extra laundry, but just as with cloth diapering, it really isn't a big deal once you get in the habit. Here are a few tips that have made things easier, though:

- Use separate loads for microfiber and towels/napkins so the microfiber doesn't pick up the lint from the others.

- Once every month or so: Run a rinse cycle with some baking soda first to cut any grease.

- Run an extra rinse cycle with vinegar at the end if needed for extra cleaning/deodorizing.

- Use natural oxy bleach occasionally to get rid of stains or odor (I also sometimes use this on cloth diapers).

- Wash every other day and teach younger kids to fold the loads (learning how to fold cloths is an easy start).

Begin switching to natural cleaning products and a paper-free kitchen. You'll save money, and if you prepare these cleaners in bulk, you'll save time too because you won't be running to the store all the time to grab what you need. And, for less than $60 you can get a good supply of all of the cloth replacements for paper products in your kitchen. Start saving today while creating a toxin-free home.

Chapter 12

improve indoor air quality

Although it doesn't get as much press, indoor air pollution has been shown to be two to five times as contaminated as outdoor air in some places, and indoor air is usually much more stagnant.

What exactly is causing the pollution? Chemical-based cleaners, air fresheners, scents, and detergents are the main culprits. These products contain harsh chemicals that wreak all kinds of havoc on the body, from eye irritation to breathing problems to reproductive damage.

Aren't you glad you're switching over to natural products?

Especially if you're just making the switch, you can use natural methods to help clean up the air inside your house. These simple ways to improve the air quality can make a big difference.

OPEN THE WINDOWS

One of the reasons indoor air can be so toxic is that it is usually very stagnant. Heating and cooling units just recirculate the same air, keeping harmful chemicals, allergens, and pollutants trapped inside the home. When weather allows, just open the windows to freshen the air. This is the easiest way to improve indoor air (assuming you don't live in the middle of a downtown area with high smog levels).

GROW PLANTS FOR CLEAN AIR

Houseplants are a natural solution to indoor air pollution. Through photosynthesis, plants take in carbon dioxide and release oxygen in its place. The plant then breaks down the gas and sends it to its roots. Microbes living in the roots of the plants use the gas and other absorbed chemicals from the air as food. Plant soils and leaves also release moisture, which helps keep indoor air humidified.

I found a short list of plants that are good at filtering indoor air, are resilient, and are considered nontoxic for children, and these are the houseplants we currently have:

- Aloe vera (*Aloe vera*), in addition to its air-filtering abilities, contains a gel in its leaves that is great for burns when topically applied.

- Spider plant (*Chlorophytum comosum*) is very resilient and produces runners (smaller plants) that can be transplanted.

- Snake plant (*Sansevieria trifasciata* 'Laurentii'), also called mother-in-law's tongue, is one of the best for filtering out formaldehyde, which is common in cleaning products, toilet paper, tissues, and personal care products.

- Dracaena (*Dracaena deremensis* 'Warneckii'), also known as corn plant, helps remove formaldehyde, which can cause respiratory problems and headaches, from the indoor environment. Formaldehyde is found in carpet backing and particleboard furniture.

- Christmas cactus (*Schlumbergera x buckleyi*) is a colorful plant that powerfully extracts chemicals from the air.

- Boston fern (*Nephrolepis exaltata*), an easy-to-grow, hardy favorite, is excellent at filtering the air.

- Bromeliads (Bromeliaceae) are tropical looking and colorful and are great air filters.

- Bamboo palm (*Chamaedorea seifrizii*), also known as the reed palm, is a small palm that thrives in shady indoor spaces. Place them near furniture that could be off-gassing formaldehyde; this plant also filters out benzene and trichloroethylene.

- Yucca (Asparagaceae). Requiring lots of light, this desert plant is good at filtering the air.

USE NATURAL AIR FILTER OPTIONS

Besides indoor plants, there are other great natural air filter options available now.

Electronic Air Filters

Look for an electronic air filter with a HEPA-type filter that is rated to remove dust, allergens, and chemicals from the air. Check out my resources page at WellnessMama.com or go to WellnessMama.com/go/air-doctor/.

Beeswax Candles

Regular paraffin candles are petroleum derived and can release chemicals like benzene, toluene, soot, and other toxins into the air. These candles do more harm than good for indoor air quality and should be avoided.

Pure beeswax candles, on the other hand, burn with almost no smoke or scent and clean the air by releasing negative ions into the air. These ions can bind with toxins and help remove them from the air.

Beeswax candles are often especially helpful for those with asthma or allergies and they are effective at removing common allergens like dust and dander from the air. They also burn more slowly than paraffin candles so they last much longer.

SALT LAMPS

Salt lamps are another natural way to clean indoor air and work as air purifiers. Made from Himalayan salt crystals, salt lamps are essentially large pieces of pure Himalayan salt with a small bulb inside. They also release negative ions into the air to help clean it and are a beautiful light source. The only downside . . . my kids like to lick them!

These soothing lamps may also help boost mood and energy levels, especially for those with seasonal affective disorder (SAD). The soft orange hues are one of the soothing colors often used to calm mood and increase focus. The small number of negative ions may also be helpful in boosting mood as well.

My brother-in-law has struggled with asthma and allergies for much of his life, and he found relief from using a Himalayan salt inhaler. Others have also noticed a difference from having salt lamps in their homes or offices.

You can also use salt lamps as a night-light. The natural orange glow doesn't disrupt sleep hormones the way fluorescent and blue lights do. And I find it very relaxing. We have an 8-inch salt lamp that we use regularly (it is also the most cost effective for its size, as the bigger lamps can get very pricey).

Salt lamps cost less than many other types of lamps, and a high-quality one can last for decades. If you are interested in adding a salt lamp to your home, choose ones with these features for best quality:

Orange Color. Darker-colored lamps are typically considered higher quality. Lamps should specify that they are 100 percent Himalayan salt, as cheap imitations may use lower quality salt.

Size. The bigger the salt lamp, the greater the effect. Smaller lamps weigh 5 to 6 pounds while larger ones can weigh up to 50 pounds. A good general rule is that 1 pound of salt will filter approximately a 4 x 4-foot area of a room. Smaller lamps are typically much less expensive, so we keep 1 to 2 in smaller rooms and 2 to 3 in larger rooms of our home.

Rough Surface. The surface quality of a salt lamp determines its "hygroscopic" potential. This describes the phenomenon of attracting and holding water molecules from the air in order to prevent dry air, which can cause dry nasal passages and sore throat symptoms. Rougher lamps have a higher surface area than smooth and polished lamps and are more effective at improving air quality. In my opinion, they also look better and are a great decoration for most rooms.

Bulb. The hygroscopic benefits result from the interaction between heat and the salt, so it is important to use a heat-producing bulb. LED bulbs don't accomplish this. I use a basic watt T6 tubular 25T6 lightbulb for Himalayan salt lamps, available from Amazon.

CHARCOAL BAGS

Activated charcoal has a natural toxin-removing effect on the air. We use bamboo charcoal in burlap bags in our house. They work wonders for odor removal and removing toxins from the air.

WHAT ARE NEGATIVE IONS?

At any given time, there are both positive and negative ions in the air. As a flashback to freshman science class:

> *An ion is an atom or molecule in which the total number of electrons is not equal to the total number of protons, giving the atom a net positive or negative electrical charge.*

Positively charged ions are also known as cations; negatively charged ions are anions. The positive or negative charge makes ions able to move and bond easily.

Negative ions occur more commonly in nature, and they are often created by lightning storms, sunlight, waterfalls, ocean waves, and so on. Running water is considered nature's greatest source of negative ions and may be one of the things that contributes to the refreshing scent of waterfalls and the beach. In fact, this is one of the reasons people often report feeling renewed or refreshed after a storm or at the beach.

WebMD explains some of the benefits of negative ions in the air:

> *"Generally speaking, negative ions increase the flow of oxygen to the brain, resulting in higher alertness, decreased drowsiness, and more mental energy," says Pierce J. Howard, PhD, author of* The Owner's Manual for the Brain: Everyday Applications from Mind Brain Research *and director of research at the Center for Applied Cognitive Sciences in Charlotte, N.C.*
>
> *"They also may protect against germs in the air, resulting in decreased irritation due to inhaling various particles that make you sneeze, cough, or have a throat irritation."*
>
> *And for the whopping one in three of us who are sensitive to their effects, negative ions can make us feel like we are walking on air. You are one of them if you feel instantly refreshed the moment you open a window and breathe in fresh, humid air.*

With a few simple tweaks, you can clear the air in your house. My suggestions should also accent your decor, so you'll not only have a pollution-free home but a well-decorated one too.

Chapter 13

clean up your home water supply

What do all of the following have in common? Making tea, washing your hands, taking a shower, and steaming veggies. All of these activities, and thousands more, require pure, unpolluted water.

Our bodies depend on water for life. It transports oxygen and nutrients to cells. It controls our body temperature. It lubricates and cushions our joints and organs. Brain function, immunity, and elimination all rely on water. Proper hydration creates youthful skin. You can live for days without food, but you will die in a few days from lack of water.

But regular tap water can have its own share of problems. If you're drinking tap water, there's a chance you're also swilling more than three hundred chemicals and pollutants, according to research from the Environmental Working Group. Among these contaminants are:

- **Arsenic.** This odorless and tasteless semi-metal element enters drinking water supplies from natural deposits, as well as agricultural and industrial wastes. Human exposure to arsenic can cause both short- and long-term health consequences, including cancer.

- **Bacteria.** Nasty pathogens from human waste and soil runoff frequently contaminate well and city water, posing a risk for serious illness upon exposure. City water is commonly derived from treated sewage.

- **Chlorine.** This free radical disinfectant can quickly damage our hair, skin, and lungs when we bathe or shower. It has also been shown to cause gastric upset upon ingestion and has been linked to malfunction of the liver and immune system with long-term exposure.

- **Chloramines.** Now being added to nearly all municipal water districts, chloramines are formed by the combination of chlorine and ammonia. Chloramines are so strong that they tend to dissolve the inside of your pipes and fixtures, releasing contaminants and heavy metals into the water. Chloramines have been linked to anemia and to liver, kidney, and central nervous system, and reproductive problems.

- **Endocrine-Disrupting Chemicals.** These are substances that may mimic or interfere with the normal hormones in the body. From this testimony before a congressional committee on the issue: "Over the past fifty years, researchers observed increases in endocrine-sensitive health outcomes. Breast and prostatic cancer incidence increased between 1969 and 1986; there was a four-fold increase in ectopic pregnancies (development of the fertilized egg outside of the uterus) in the U.S. between 1970 and 1987; the incidence of cryptorchidism (undescended testicles) doubled in the U.K. between 1960 and the mid-1980s; and there was an approximately 42% decrease in sperm count worldwide between 1940 and 1990."

- **Fluoride.** Many communities receive pre-treated, fluoridated water in their homes. Fluoride, known as "the devil's poison," has been shown to be less than effective in preventing tooth decay while possibly contributing to a whole host of health concerns, such as thyroid problems when consumed internally.

- **Gasoline.** Easily absorbed into the soil, even a small gas spill or leak can contaminate groundwater sources. Considered a hazardous waste material, consumption has significant adverse effects on the central nervous system.

- **Hardness.** Hard water is the result of calcium and magnesium present in the water. These minerals form white scale buildup creating problems for water heaters, washing machines, dishwashers, and plumbing systems. This condition creates a lack of lather when using soap and can contribute to dingy laundry.

- **Heavy Metals.** These include lead and mercury, which have been linked to many health problems.

- **Pesticides and Herbicides.** These can contaminate groundwater, well water aquifers, and city water reserves. Exposure has been linked to chronic illness, birth defects, and weakened immunity.

- **Radon.** This is a harmful radioactive gas sometimes found in drinking water and indoor air. Exposure to radon increases cancer risk, particularly lung cancer.

WHAT TO DRINK?

Drinking plenty of pure water throughout the day is vital for boosting the body's detoxification powers. The best option is to drink filtered or high-quality bottled spring water (from glass bottles). Water that provides additional electrolytes such as calcium, potassium, and magnesium is also a good choice, especially if you sweat quite a bit or have lost water through exercise.

For many families, a water filter is a cost-effective way to have clean water at all times. There are many great options available, but look for one that removes most or all of the contaminants listed above. If you want to see the ones my family uses, go to wellnessmama .com/8079/water-filter-options/.

CHEMICALS IN BATHWATER

In the 1990s, the EPA acknowledged that a person can absorb more chlorine and other contaminants from bath and shower water than even from drinking water polluted with the same substances.

Unfortunately, this puts children most at risk, because some children bathe for forty-five minutes or more several nights a week. Because children also have a larger surface area to body weight ratio, they may absorb chemicals more quickly and be more severely affected by them.

Children's tissues, organs, and biological systems are still developing, with several stages of rapid growth and development occurring from infancy to adolescence. This rapid development, combined with the immaturity of body organs and systems, predisposes children to potentially more severe consequences within certain age ranges and windows of vulnerability.

Most municipal water supplies use chlorine to help reduce the number of pathogens in the water. Unfortunately, the cure can sometimes be as bad as the disease!

When chlorine is used to treat water, it combines with organic matter in the water to create compounds called trihalomethanes (THMs). These are essentially by-products of the disinfection process. One of the most common THMs formed is chloroform, a known carcinogen. Other types of THMs formed include di- and trichloramines formed when chloramine is used as a disinfecting agent. These compounds are considered toxic when consumed, inhaled, or applied to the skin. Carbon block filters will remove chlorine and chloramines, but they can be tough to use for bath or shower water. One of the easiest ways to rapidly improve bathwater is to add a little vitamin C. This vitamin is great for the immune system, but it can also play a role in reducing the chemicals in bath water.

Two forms of vitamin C work to neutralize chlorine: sodium ascorbate and ascorbic acid. Personally, I prefer to use the sodium ascorbate form because it has less of an effect on the pH of the water, but both work.

Just 1 teaspoon of either sodium ascorbate or ascorbic acid should be enough to neutralize a tub of water. It is best to add the powder 2 to 5 minutes before getting in the bath to allow it to work.

When you are educated about what you drink and how it affects you, you can make significant but simple lifestyle changes to drastically improve your health. Water is life giving . . . as long as it's pure and toxin-free.

Our smartphones, tablets, computers, and related digital devices have become so important to us that they have changed life as we used to know it.

But how much is too much? Or, more specifically, how many of us have the nagging feeling that we somehow can't disconnect from the devices we own because those devices have begun to own us? And how are they affecting our health and our relationships?

If you believe, like I do, that we ought to spend less time checking and rechecking our many screens and instead spend more time taking part in real life, maybe it's time for a digital detox. Here are some of the best ways to find balance between screen time and face time.

Welcome to Step 4!

Chapter 14

try a technological fast

Everyone seems to be glued to their smartphones, computers, or tablets these days. If I go out with my friends, at least one of us is constantly on the phone. That's crazy!

Is this "can't live without" piece of technology a godsend in our increasingly fast-paced world? Or are we wired for trouble?

Some startling statistics reflect how technology affects our lives:

- One third of families feel smartphones are disruptive at the dinner table, and one in three people has argued with his or her partner about mobile phone use.

- The average person reaches for her smartphone 100 to 200 times a day.

- One-third of women who use social media log on to Facebook the second they wake up.

Wow. Besides the fact that technology seems to be constantly in the way, it also may be shortening attention span. Remember the days when you (or your kids) used to spend hours engrossed in a book? Or read the daily newspaper from top to bottom? Now we're headfirst into our computer screens with dozens of open tabs, simultaneously skimming the news, scrolling Facebook feeds, and checking our emails.

Some neuroscientists believe that these habits have left us with "neural fatigue." Our brains are so busy absorbing facts, pseudo-facts, and jibber-jabber all posing as information that it's hard to stay focused on anything longer than a tweet.

All of this crazy processing increases the stress hormone cortisol, which further scrambles our ability to think clearly. And information overload, nonstop distractions, and high-pressure schedules all take a toll on our mood, stress level, and relationships.

Admittedly. though, I can't imagine what I'd do without my cell phone. And I confess that when I'm sitting free somewhere, I'm checking my apps, looking at Facebook, reading emails, or mindlessly googling something. Often, I feel like a slave to the tech age!

There's no question that technology makes our lives better, but I feel like it might be having a negative impact on our family ties and on our lives. In addition to living a more natural life in terms of food, exercise, and home remedies, I began to reflect on the way my own family relates digitally. Yes, it's vital to detox from nutrition-barren foods, toxins, and stress and to exercise more, but perhaps we should pay closer attention to how we relate to those around us.

But where does our relationship—notice the term—with technology come into all of this? Did I need to assess how much time I spend on my smartphone and other mobile devices? Did I need a digital detox from the constant stream of texts, emails, notifications, and reminders on those devices so that I could reconnect to the world around me? The answers for me were yes, so I—along with my family—took a technological fast, and I'd encourage you to try one too, especially if you feel like you're a bit addicted to your phone, computer, tablet, or the Internet in general.

DON'T GO COLD TURKEY

I would never recommend that anyone get rid of their devices or technology. It's all about bal-ance. For example, instead of checking Twitter, Facebook, and email as soon as you get up, take a few moments to go through your morning routine: work out, eat breakfast, send your kids off to school—whatever you do to "start" your day. Take time to do it and then jump into your emails and social accounts.

CUT BACK GRADUALLY

If the urge to check your phone is habitual, build up to a stage where you only need to check your phone a couple of times a day. Start by proving to yourself that you can go a half hour without it, then an hour, then two.

SET SOME RULES AND STICK TO THEM

Create some rules: No Facebook after 6 p.m., Instagram on weekends only, or no Twitter at work. If you're an "oversharer," try posting photos weekly instead of daily or updating your status less frequently during the week.

RETHINK YOUR APPS

Having Facebook, Twitter, and email on your phone or computer's home screen (or even having your browser open them all right away) may seem like a good idea, but it actually stops you from being productive. Set a time to scan your feeds (or apps) at the top of every hour or every other hour, depending on your personal and professional needs. Hide the apps on your home screen in a special folder, or perhaps move them to the second screen. Set up Twitter notifications for specific accounts so you don't have to worry about missing that one crucial tweet.

ENGAGE IN FUN NON-TECHIE ACTIVITIES

Instead of getting on your phone, get outside and walk in nature at least once a week, or go to the gym. Develop a meditation practice that you can manage in your life.

SEE REAL FRIENDS

Social media was developed to increase connections among people, even despite geographic distances. It has helped create communities of people with similar interests or beliefs, and it's reconnected us with people we otherwise wouldn't be able to see. It can provide educational opportunities and enhance technical skills. These are all potential benefits, but risks exist as well.

The more time you spend on social networking sites, the less time you have to hang out with friends and family in person. And online interactions are missing the richest parts of relationships. Make it a point to spend more time with friends—and not through their Instagram feed. Meet for coffee or meals, take classes together, or find exercise buddies.

MAKE REGULAR DEVICE-FREE PLANS

You might try leaving your phone in the car while you shop or dine out, or put your phone on airplane mode. Make certain times of the day technology-free zones. Bedtime and mealtimes are easy places to start—why not try making the hours between 6 and 8 p.m. phone-free family time? Or try a technology-free day at the weekend, if you can. Respond to emails and texts only at specific times of the day. Pick three times—say, 9 a.m., 1 p.m., and 4 p.m.—and check your messages only then. Turn off email and social media notifications, or turn down your volume settings to reduce the urge to constantly check mobile devices.

Hopefully you too will find that you can control technology instead of letting technology control you.

Chapter 15

guide your kids on digital life

When my husband and I take our family out to eat in a restaurant, it saddens me to see kids who once they sit down flip out their iPads or smartphones at the dinner table. They're so busy with technology that they can't possibly spend quality time with their family, or enjoy conversation, sharing, and laughter.

Digital exposure as a whole is on the rise, with one study indicating that the average eight- to ten-year-old spends almost eight hours per day on social media, while preteens and teenagers spend more than eleven hours per day. All of this screen time brings on health problems. Take a look:

Weight Gain. Kids glued to their tablets, smartphones, or computers for hours on end may be more likely to become obese, suggests research from Illinois State University. Researchers asked more than seven hundred kids to wear pedometers (to gauge how much they moved around), plus report on how much time they spent watching TV and playing video games. The researchers found the greater the kids' screen time, the less they exercised and the more weight they gained.

Risky Behaviors. Canadian researchers found that young people who spent more than three or four hours a day at their computers were 50 percent more likely to engage in risky behaviors such as drinking, smoking, drug use, and unprotected sex than kids who spend a minimal amount of time at the computer. Why was this? The researchers suggested that kids who use computers can be regularly exposed to many examples of dangerous behaviors, which they may then emulate.

Psychological Health. Tellingly, the more time teenagers spend using a computer or watching TV, the weaker their emotional bonds are with their parents. That's the conclusion of a study of more than three thousand teens published in the *Archives of Pediatrics & Adolescent Medicine*. On the other hand, teens who spent more time reading and doing homework reported feeling closer to their moms and dads. The researchers noted that when kids feel a healthful attachment to their parents, this boosts psychological health and reduces participation in risky health behaviors.

There's an upside to gadgets, however. They can help our kids grow and learn. There are lots of educational and creative apps and programs that can be downloaded to challenge children's creativity. When your kid is concentrating on a game, for example, he or she is actually improving mental capacity. In experiments comparing "gamers" to "nongamers," scientists discovered that frequent players (gamers) have sharper vision and faster reaction times and that they're better at multitasking and have better concentration than nongamers.

As for cell phones, they are great for safety and peace of mind for us parents. When kids are out with friends, the cell phone can be a lifeline in case of an emergency.

As parents, we need to be mindful of what our kids share online and what they may choose to post. We may think we can't live without our technology, and to a certain extent we can't in our increasingly fast-paced world. However, I think kids need a digital detox too. If your kids and teens are head down over their electronic devices or glued to their games more than you'd like, it might be a good idea to set some boundaries and guidelines.

ENCOURAGE NONDIGITAL ACTIVITIES

When your kids are playing electronic games all the time, they aren't getting much fresh air. They're not reading books, having face-to-face interactions with peers, or playing creatively. Videos, computers, apps, and portable games are here to stay, but let's not forget the value of simple play outdoors with bicycling, ball games, and other physical activities.

Also, getting your kids involved in after-school activities, whether sports, dance, music, or art, helps reduce too much online interaction.

KEEP TABS ON KIDS' ONLINE ACTIVITY

It's important to screen social media use, both in terms of time spent and types of sites visited. Actively monitor usage and set limits on time used. Consider establishing a maximum time that may be spent on social media in a single day, or insist on shutting off all electronic devices after a certain time. Have talks with your kids about what they encounter online, and openly discuss what types of sites are and are not considered acceptable.

Also, keep computers in an open part of your home (like a kitchen workstation). That way, you can check on what your kids are doing online and how much time they are spending there.

STRESS REAL RELATIONSHIPS

Kids need to be taught that the most meaningful conversations take place face-to-face—which is why it's a good idea to limit the use of digital devices. It's important for kids to be connected to people and family members and not just isolated in their own rooms. Social media is great, but you also have to get out there and interact with people.

SET EXPECTATIONS

As a parent, it's your responsibility to determine how and when devices can be used: only *x* number of texts a day, for example, or no social media during homework or during dinner. Mealtimes are important occasions to really connect with one another without the technological distractions that can be so overwhelming throughout the day.

Some families insist that all children's laptops and cell phones must be in charge mode in the kitchen during overnight hours. Others make a rule that cell phones must be turned off by 10 p.m. Basically, our goal as parents is to help our children develop a healthful relationship with technology.

HELP YOUR KIDS BE SAFE ONLINE

Make it clear to your kids that online interactions should be limited to only people they know and that personal information should not be shared without first talking to you. And encourage them to speak up to you if they feel harassed by anyone online.

Talk to them about the serious consequences of online bullying. If your child is the victim of cyberbullying, take action with the other parents and with the school, if appropriate. Attend to your kids' emotional needs promptly if they are being bullied online, and consider taking them off social media sites where the bullying occurs.

The digital world can be a wonderful place for learning. But it also is a place where kids can run into trouble. Make sure kids of all ages know that it is inappropriate to send or receive pictures of people without clothing or sexy text messages.

"Friend" your kids on social media sites they use. That way, you can monitor their online presence.

Don't hesitate to use parental controls. They're a useful tool in the effort to ensure responsible usage. Most smartphones and laptops come with either built-in controls or easy-to-download apps that can help parents control how, what, and when their child uses his or her new gadget.

CREATE A PERSONALIZED MEDIA PLAN

Check out the link HealthyChildren.org/Media UsePlan. It helps you create a personalized Family Media Use Plan that works within your family's values and busy lifestyles.

This interactive tool developed by the American Academy of Pediatrics (AAP) includes a Media Time Calculator that can give you a snapshot of how much time your kids are spending on such activities as sleeping, eating, doing homework, exercising, and using social media. It also includes AAP recommendations on screen-free zones, media manners, and much more.

Remember that your kids are watching you, so it's important to set a good example with your own digital usage. If you're engaging your child in conversation, then don't pull out your phones and start texting—you wouldn't let your child do that to you. We have to remember that as adults, it's our responsibility to be great role models for our children.

Six children, a business to run, and tight deadlines often leave me frazzled and in desperate need of some time out. Over the years, I've discovered three powerful allies in my "war" on stress: spending time in nature, exercising, and detoxing my sleep habits. All three can help you think more positively and bring about a heightened sense of well-being and relaxation—and can work for the entire family.

Welcome to Step 5!

Chapter 16

find your path to the outdoors

There is a whole world outside, so what is keeping us indoors? Sadly, it's the usual culprits, namely, time constraints and our "need" to stay glued to our computers, tablets, phones, and TVs. So it's no wonder people hesitate to spend a day outdoors! But let's reconsider, so we don't miss out on all the beauty and restorative power that nature offers.

Science is now on the side of nature, the outdoors, and those who love being outside. In fact, there is a term for the health-boosting, stress-relieving value of nature—*ecotherapy*, which refers to the various physical and psychological benefits of being outside.

A 2009 study found that the closer someone lived to a green space or nature area, the healthier that person was likely to be. In fact, those who lived closest to a park, nature preserve, or wooded area were less likely to suffer from anxiety or depression.

Another study found that those who spent time hiking or resting in a forest had measurably lower cortisol (stress hormone) rates, heart rates, and blood pressure.

The University of Illinois conducted research that showed that children with ADD/ADHD experienced a reduction of symptoms after spending time outdoors (this ties in with a less well-studied theory that these disorders are at least partially "nature-deficit disorders"). Of course, just spending time in nature won't be a silver bullet for children struggling with ADD/ADHD, but spending some (free!) family time outdoors is worth a try.

Other studies have found sleep improvements, better immune system function, and lower rates of stress-related disorders in those who spent regular time in nature.

So why is nature so important?

VITAMIN D

One reason time outdoors may contribute to health is the exposure to vitamin D–producing sunlight. This vital prehormone (a substance later converted to an active hormone) is responsible for many aspects of health throughout the body. Vitamin D deficiency has been linked to various types of cancer and obesity, as well as mental disorders and other health problems. Though supplemental vitamin D is available, some people (like me) don't absorb it effectively and must obtain vitamin D through adequate sun exposure. Spending time outdoors in moderate sun is a great way to get natural vitamin D.

EXERCISE

Most nature experiences also include some form of exercise—the greatest stress-busting activity ever. Whether rock climbing, swimming, hiking, or canoeing, most forms of outdoor activity also include movement. Spending time outdoors provides a chance for fun movement along with the other benefits of nature. Since we should all be moving each day anyway, get the double benefit and get your exercise outdoors!

GETTING GROUNDED

"Grounding" is based on the theory that since many of us don't come into direct skin contact with the earth very often, a positive charge can build up in the body.

Direct skin contact with the earth acts as a "ground" just like it does for electrical outlets, reducing this extra positive charge. Propo-

nents of grounding report that it helps reduce inflammation in the body, relieves stress, and improves sleep quality.

You can practice grounding by walking barefoot, gardening, strolling on the beach, or swimming in a natural body of water.

If you can't get outdoors, you can still obtain the benefits of grounding by using special "earthing mats" or "sheets."

FRESH AIR

Indoor air is up to seventy times more contaminated than outdoor air. With more airtight insulation, windows and doors, and the plethora of chemicals and plastics we bring into our homes, most people come in contact with up to six thousand chemicals regularly.

Spending time outdoors provides a break from indoor air pollution, and outdoor air may have additional benefits as well. Outdoor air is a good source of beneficial negative ions. Negative ions are referred to as "nature's antidepressants" and are found to have a relaxing and healing effect. Being at the beach and near waterfalls are especially good ways to connect to these ions. Negative ions are also present in sunlight. After a thunderstorm, you can smell the "freshness" in the air. Indoor air, by contrast, is deficient in negative ions and is often dry and contaminated.

EYE HEALTH

Better eye health is a surprising benefit of spending time outdoors, and an increasingly important one. Our society is seeing an increase in vision problems, especially in children. One possible reason is the amount of time that many of us spend looking at a computer or TV screen on a daily basis.

While children used to spend most of their time outdoors, looking at a wide variety of colors, levels of brightness, and depths, they now spend up to seven hours a day staring at a TV, computer, or tablet screen with artificial light. The result is an increase in nearsightedness, even in kids who aren't genetically predisposed to it.

In fact, a study done in 2007 found that children who spent at least two hours a day outside were four times less likely to be nearsighted. For children, this has especially dire consequences. The researchers speculated that bright outdoor light helps children develop the correct distance between retina and lens and leads to better eyesight later in life. Since indoor lighting does not provide the same benefit, children who spend a lot of time indoors are much more likely to have vision problems later in life.

Staring at a screen can also lead to eye fatigue, headaches, neck and back problems, and other problems in adults.

WEIGHT LOSS

Need to drop some pounds? Spend more time outdoors, especially in morning sunlight. In fact, a study at Northwestern University found that the earlier a study participant got morning sunlight, the lower the participant's BMI. This correlation remained strong even after researchers adjusted for exercise levels, age, calorie intake, and other factors that affect your weight. The reason? Getting sunlight in the morning helps keep cortisol levels and circadian rhythms in the right ranges.

The reverse correlation was also true, as exposure to light at night was a factor in gaining weight (another reason to make sure you have a dark sleep environment), but as little as half an hour of sun exposure before noon was enough to have an effect on reducing body weight. This effect is so pronounced, in fact, that my doctor recommended morning sunlight exposure as part of my protocol to help improve my cortisol levels and thyroid health.

Does indoor light work?

Bright morning light outdoors is typically thousands of "lux," a measure of illuminance that is essentially one lumen per square meter. Indoor light typically only measures a few hundred lux and doesn't contain the broad spectrum of light needed to correctly support the body's internal clock.

While 10,000 lux energy light lamps get closer to the level of outdoor brightness and are often used in the winter by those who suffer from SAD, nothing beats the benefits of nature with true sunshine.

Walking in Nature

I love taking long morning walks on a greenway near our home where there are plenty of trees, wildflowers, and even a small waterfall. I sometimes take my children on these walks, and I always encourage them to spend time outdoors in the morning as well. Whatever works for you, find a way to spend some time outdoors each day and take your family with you.

LET THEM GET DIRTY

Thanks to modern hygiene and sanitation, we've experienced lower rates of many diseases and health problems. Unfortunately, too much of a good thing can have its problems. Gardeners (statistically) live longer, and it turns out that the dirt itself plays a role here. You see, the clean life may throw off the delicate balance of our immune systems. And that's why today, you get to start loosening some rules on your family's relationship to dirt.

MODERN HYGIENE'S DIRTY TRICKS

We all need healthy gut bacteria. Restoring this beneficial bacteria could be the key to boosting immune function, reducing rates of allergies or digestive problems, and even improving mood.

So where are these healthy bacteria and how can we benefit from them?

Sure, you can take probiotic-rich foods and supplements. But if you really want to round out your healthy intake of probiotics, look to soil-based organisms (SBOs), found in the soil. Exposure to SBOs in the dirt is good for immunity.

For centuries, various cultures have known the health benefits of dirt. There is an old saying that "you have to eat a peck of dirt before you die." It seems there is wisdom in this old saying. As this 2009 article in the *New York Times* explains:

In studies of what is called the hygiene hypothesis, researchers are concluding that organisms like the millions of bacteria, viruses and especially worms that enter the body along with "dirt" spur the development of a healthy immune system. Several continuing studies suggest that worms may help to redirect an immune system that has gone awry and resulted in autoimmune disorders, allergies and asthma.

These studies, along with epidemiological observations, seem to explain why immune system disorders like multiple sclerosis, Type 1 diabetes, inflammatory bowel disease, asthma and allergies have risen significantly in the United States and other developed countries.

Heather (from the popular blog Mommypotamus) has talked about the benefits of these types of organisms for people with IBS or digestive disorders:

In [a] double-blind, placebo controlled study researchers found that IBS patients who took a soil-based probiotic experienced a significant reduction in symptoms after two weeks. A follow-up study found that the patients were still experiencing these benefits one year after discontinuing the probiotic, presumably because the beneficial bacteria stay in the gut and continue to function.

There's also a link between gut health and mental health, and it turns out that certain SBOs play an important role here too:

Mary O'Brien, an oncologist at Royal Marsden Hospital in London, first stumbled upon these findings while inoculating lung cancer patients with a strain of M. vaccae (pronounced "em vah-kay") [which is a bacteria in the dirt] to see if their symptoms improved. She noticed that in addition to fewer cancer symptoms, patients also demonstrated an improvement in emotional health, vitality, and even cognitive function. (Annals of Oncology 15 (June 2004): 906–14).

WHY DIRT IS IMPORTANT FOR KIDS

So what does it all mean for our kids? It means that all of our cleaning, disinfecting, and sterilizing could be doing more harm than good at times. Much to the chagrin of their mothers (and my husband!), babies have a natural desire to play in the dirt and put dirty objects in their mouths. Turns out, this could have an important immune-developing purpose: "What a child is doing when he puts things in his mouth is allowing his immune response to explore his environment," Mary Ruebush, a microbiology and immunology instructor, wrote in her book, *Why Dirt Is Good*. "Not only does this allow for 'practice' of immune responses, which will be necessary for protection, but it also plays a critical role in teaching the immature immune response what is best ignored."

After a study found that kids who grew up on farms or with a dog in the house had fewer allergies, research started to explore the importance of the organisms found in these less-than-sanitized environments and how they impacted health. One leading researcher, Dr. Joel V. Weinstock, the director of gastroenterology and hepatology at Tufts Medical Center in Boston, said in an interview that the immune system at birth "is like an unprogrammed computer. It needs instruction." Public health measures like cleaning up contaminated water and food have saved the lives of countless children, but they "also eliminated exposure to many organisms that are probably good for us." He continued: Children raised in an ultra-clean environment are not being exposed to organisms that help them develop appropriate immune regulatory circuits.

Dr. David Elliott, a gastroenterologist and immunologist at the University of Iowa with whom Weinstock has collaborated, noted in an interview that intestinal worms, which have been all but eliminated in developed countries, are "likely to be the biggest player" in proper immune system regulation. He added that bacterial and viral infections seem to influence the immune system in the same way, but not as forcefully.

The results of the study *American Journal of Respiratory and Critical Care Medicine* published in 2007 shows the use of cleaning sprays four times a week caused an increase in asthma. Sprays that were included in the increase in asthma were glass-cleaning, furniture, and air-freshening sprays.

WHY DIRT IS ESPECIALLY IMPORTANT FOR BABIES

The natural organisms in dirt serve an important purpose for people of all ages, but babies have a specific and additional need for interaction with dirt. Breast milk lacks iron because pathogens like *E. coli* (which can cause severe digestive problems in newborns) need iron to thrive, as do other pathogens. These low iron levels can help protect newborns from these bacteria.

Around six months, a baby's need for iron and other nutrients ramps up, but breast milk doesn't increase its levels of these nutrients, and with good reason. At this stage in life, babies spend more time on the ground. In the past, this meant they spent more time interacting with dirt, which is a good source of iron and minerals such as zinc, magnesium, and others. Iron is particularly important for preventing cognitive, motor, and behavioral deficits that may last into the teen years.

But can't your child obtain enough iron from breast milk? Not really. The Institute of Medicine recommends that infants 6 to 12 months old get 11 mg of iron per day. This iron should come from supplementary foods, in addition to breast milk or formula. You can't really meet your baby's requirement for iron on breast milk by itself. If you did, your infant would have to drink between 4 and 13 liters of breast milk a day. That's a lot!

So breast milk is inadequate? Hardly . . .

All this research shows that babies are capable of absorbing iron from soil (which they are naturally in contact with at this age if playing on the ground). Other mammals have breast milk that is naturally low in iron at the same developmental times and these mammals are also capable of absorbing iron and other nutrients from the soil, indicating that there is a biological reason for this.

In the past, the umbilical cord also wasn't clamped immediately after birth (and there is good reason to delay clamping it these days too), which allowed more of the umbilical cord blood (the baby's blood) to flow into the baby. This resulted in higher iron levels, which would also help baby maintain iron levels for a longer time.

HOW TO MAKE SURE WE GET ENOUGH DIRT

- Go outside more often.

- Eat some dirt. Just kidding! We don't actually need to make an effort to consume dirt to get the benefits of SBOs and nutrients in soil—we just need to make an effort to come in contact with it (along with our babies and children).

- Encourage your kids (including crawling babies) to play outside barefoot in the dirt as long as the area hasn't been sprayed with chemicals or contaminated in some other way. Spend time in the garden and walk outside barefoot.

- Let your babies have an outside play area with organic dirt once they are three to four months or old enough to sit up or crawl. This area can be just a small kiddie pool or even a pot of organic dirt with some toys in it to encourage play. Yes, the babies get dirty. Yes, they put it in their mouths (that is the point).

- Have your older kids help you in the garden and with yard work. Encourage them to play in the dirt too. If they've been playing in clean dirt, I also let mine eat outside without washing their hands so they can transfer small amounts of SBOs to their digestive systems.

- Consume fermented drinks and food like water kefir, homemade sauerkraut, and kombucha to make sure you're exposed to a wide variety of naturally occurring beneficial bacteria.

- Supplement with a high-quality probiotic/prebiotic blend that contains many of these same organisms. I also sprinkle soil-based probiotics on the foods I feed my little ones and even dump a capsule into the play dirt.

There is just so much benefit to enjoying the great outdoors and playing outside, from a healthier body to stress reduction to stronger immune function.

Chapter 17

develop a passion for exercise

Exercise is a touchy subject for a lot of people these days, but it is one of the better ways to relieve stress (not to mention, protecting your health). Some studies point out that it's more effective at boosting moods than antidepressants and antianxiety drugs.

Everyone has preferred types of exercise (from none at all to excessive and everything in between). What is truly the best type of exercise? Is it different for men and women? What about moms like me who don't have the time to log the suggested sixty minutes a day?

I'm going to answer those questions and more—and give you some fitness options you've probably never considered before. But first, here's a little background on how I came to these fitness solutions and why.

Exercise was a passion I had to develop. I wanted my kids to enjoy physical movement too and stay in shape without ever having to go "work out." (I've never liked that term! If we associate it with work, who wants to do it?) Before you can determine the best fitness program, you've got to figure out your goals. Do you just want to lose weight? Do you want to be able to compete in marathons and races? Boost cardio fitness?

My fitness goals are to release stress; have a healthy physique; be able to join a pickup game of flag football; kayak with my husband; keep up with my kids; and become strong enough to rock climb, swim, scuba dive, or hike. As a mom, a more important goal is to have the ability to react quickly and competently if a life-threatening situation ever arises, especially involving my children.

From conversations with other mothers, this last goal seems to be an important one. I know of a mom who had to crawl out a second-story window and onto her roof while holding her newborn to escape a flood. I know a mom who climbed a tree while holding a toddler to avoid an angry dog. I know a mom who jumped into a lake at a local park and swam to shore, towing a two-hundred-pound man who was having difficulty. Could I do these things? I often wonder.

While these circumstances are rare, other situations in which proper fitness determines our ability to save our own lives are much more commonplace. How many studies have you read about the links between high fitness levels and decreased risk of cancer, heart disease, and stroke?

FUNCTIONAL FITNESS IS OUR ULTIMATE GOAL

To achieve our personal exercise goals, including stress relief, I don't think that hour a day of mindless running on a treadmill like a caged hamster has a tremendous effect on survival ability. What we truly need is functional fitness—a level of fitness that makes daily activities (and more extreme ones) easier and our bodies more stress resilient. Following are three ways to develop that kind of body.

1. Short-Burst, High-Intensity Exercise

Your body has two types of muscle fibers, slow twitch and fast twitch. Slow twitch is responsible for distance and endurance at slower paces, and fast twitch is responsible for the ability to achieve short bursts of very high levels of activity. The fast-twitch fibers are actually broken into two types—fast and superfast. Regular fast-twitch fibers move approximately

five times as fast as slow-twitch fibers, and superfast-twitch fibers move about ten times as fast as slow-twitch fibers. As an example, most marathoners have about 80 percent slow twitch, while most sprinters have about 80 percent fast twitch.

According to research, most people have relatively equal levels of the two types, and this is at least partially determined by genetics. Which type of twitch fiber you work to develop will of course depend on your fitness goals, but in general, which one is better to focus on?

To answer that, I've got to talk about human growth hormone. Kids are naturally full of it, and it contributes to their rapid growth and faster ability to heal. As we get older, our levels of growth hormone decrease, and we age. Some people go so far as to spend astronomical amounts of money to receive injections of growth hormone. Where am I going with this? High-intensity exercise (short, fast bursts) has been shown to release exercise-induced growth hormone into the body. Because growth hormone is perhaps the best fat-burning, antiaging, strength-building substance we know of, it might be a good idea to get some of that kind of exercise.

The average person performing cardio at the recommended rates has about 40 percent slow-twitch fibers, 50 percent fast-twitch fibers, and 10 percent superfast-twitch fibers (not much growth hormone there!). A person who trains in high-intensity exercises has 40 percent slow-twitch fibers, 20 percent fast-twitch fibers, and 40 percent superfast-twitch fibers. That is four times the amount of growth hormone produced from exercise!

It gets better. Research shows that exercise that uses fast-twitch and superfast-twitch fibers also develops the slow-twitch fibers as well as exercise that just focuses on slow-twitch (like the treadmill). Unfortunately, the reverse is not true: Endurance exercise develops the slow-twitch fibers but does not work the fast- or superfast-twitch fibers at all (no growth hormone here!). Even worse, these fast-twitch fibers will eventually atrophy if they aren't used.

Ever see a kid younger than five logging a quick four miles before school? Kids are the experts in sprinting, climbing, and short bursts of activity that develop the growth hormone they need and produce so well. Kids do not naturally gravitate to long-distance exercise or extended patterns of the same movement over and over. How many of us could squat down for five minutes straight while playing with LEGOs? Could we climb a tree? Dominate at a game of capture the flag? What if we could maintain this level of athletic ability?

So while kids get to play outside, sprint barefoot, and climb trees, we sullenly trudge off to the gym each day to log our miles and pat ourselves on the back for our commitment to health. But if you could accomplish the same thing in thirty minutes of high-intensity exercise and use the extra ninety minutes for something else you enjoy, wouldn't you do it?

Luckily, fast-twitch and superfast-twitch fibers are developed by short bursts of high intensity of any type of exercise. For some, this may be running sprints; for others, riding a spin bike; and for others still, lifting kettlebells. As long as it is fast and short, it will work. Personally, I just head outside and sprint it out, but I know a lot of people who, because of previous injuries or bad knees, get their sprints in on a bike and have great results. I was able to run

a sprint triathlon (technically an endurance-type event) after training almost entirely with high-intensity activity in short bursts. I barely endurance-trained at all and was able to run, swim, and bike faster than I ever had. I did weight training (mainly kettlebells) to develop strength and can actually do a pull-up now, a feat I previously thought impossible!

NUTRITIONAL POWER FOR EXERCISE

There are a few other factors, of course, that contribute to the success of this type of exercise. Emerging research shows that consuming fructose (even from fruit) within two hours of a high-intensity exercise releases the chemical somatostatin in the body, effectively stopping growth hormone production. Eating an extremely high-fat meal within an hour before a workout can also inhibit growth hormone production.

Removing grains from your diet and consuming the right kinds of fats and proteins will also allow your body to increase fast-twitch fiber, improve athletic performance, and burn body fat more quickly. Getting enough sleep, drinking enough water, and obtaining enough vitamin D are also crucial.

2. Sprints

Twice a week, I do sprint sets. I use a modified Tabata routine interspersed with a longer rest routine. It looks something like this:

- Sprint 20 seconds.
- Rest 10 seconds.
- Repeat above two steps eight times.

Then:

- Sprint 30 seconds.
- Rest 60 seconds.
- Repeat above two steps eight times.

Then:

- Sprint 20 seconds.
- Rest 10 seconds.
- Repeat above two steps eight times.

You can do these by running, riding a stationary bike, lifting kettlebells, or performing any other activity that can be done quickly. I don't recommend swimming for sprints because it doesn't give you the benefits of weight-bearing exercise.

3. Strength Training

To be functionally fit, you've got to be strong. Strength training—moving your body against resistance—gets you there. I'm a big propo-nent of strength training because it can be done anywhere, relative to your fitness level, and you can do it using your body weight. This is less likely to cause injury than free weights might (especially if weights are done using poor form!).

Body-weight exercises can also be done quickly and without any added equipment, making them perfect for a workout while your kids are napping. Two or three times a week, I incorporate about twenty minutes' worth each time I strength-train, working up to more, or starting with less as needed. I focus primarily on the following exercises:

- Pull-Ups. These can be done on a tree branch or a portable pull-up bar in a doorframe. Start with assisted pull-ups if needed.

- Push-Ups. Build up your strength with wall push-ups or modified (knees on the ground) push-ups. Work up to doing them with your feet elevated on a bench or in a handstand.

- Squats. Start easy if you need to and work up to a full, deep squat.

- Planks. One of the best all-over exercises you can do. Support your plank with forearms and toes. Hold for as long as possible. Repeat several times. Once you can do this, mix it up by raising one arm or leg and holding the position or by holding in a low-push-up position instead of resting on forearms.

I'm not a doctor or even a personal trainer, so of course you should consult with yours before beginning any exercise routine.

Chapter 18

detox your sleeping habits

My husband and I met during a trekking vacation, with the goal of walking across America. During this adventure, we didn't have much time to sleep. "We'll sleep when we're dead," we often said. Turns out, not getting enough sleep can make that day come sooner that we expect! Lack of adequate sleep (six to eight hours a night) has been linked to many health problems. (See "Health Consequences of Chronic Sleeplessness" on page 112.)

While it seems like common sense that we all need adequate sleep, statistics show again and again that we just aren't getting it. For some (including me), the idea of ever getting a solid night of uninterrupted sleep again may sound wonderful, but it sure can be unrealistic. My excuse is the constant presence of a child under eighteen months in my house, but for many others it is insomnia, sleep disturbances, or simply not enough time.

I've got some detox-your-sleep-habits strategies to help you. Some you may have tried; some may be entirely new. Select several of these strategies and start applying them to your "sleepytime" right away.

SET UP A SLEEP-CONDUCIVE BEDROOM

We spend about one-third of our life sleeping, so it's important to make sure that your sleep environment promotes quality sleep and health in as many ways as possible. By improving your sleep, you'll enhance your physical health, mental focus, and even work performance. Following are some tips that can make a tremendous difference.

HEALTH CONSEQUENCES OF CHRONIC SLEEPLESSNESS

Impaired memory and higher incidence of accidents

Weakened immune system

Increased cancer risk and accelerated tumor growth

Blood sugar problems and a prediabetic state

Impaired cognitive and physical function

Reduced nerve cell generation

Increased incidence of depression

Increased inflammation in the body

Cardiovascular stress

Brain shrinkage

Impaired kidney function

Increased risk of diabetes and obesity

Increased instance of heart disease

Infertility

ADHD and behavioral problems in children

Lose the Light!

Light, or lack thereof, is vital for regulating circadian rhythm and sleep patterns. The presence of even a small amount of blue light from electronic devices and television in the bedroom at night can reduce levels of melatonin (the sleep hormone) and disrupt your sleep. This aspect of getting a good night's sleep is so important that I wear dorky orange sunglasses at night, which protect me from any ambient light, and I cover the blue light on my smoke alarm with electrical tape.

Many of us assume we're sleeping in darkness, but we forget to consider the light emitted from our clocks, charging cell phones, and TV cable boxes, just to name a few sources.

Why do these matter so much? Throughout much of human history, we had sunlight during the day and no light or only orange hues from the moon, stars, or campfire at night. Now we have artificial light in various shades and spectrums, and our bodies respond to each one differently. Even ambient light in a normal house is twelve to thirty times brighter than natural moonlight and in much different colors.

At night, in darkness, our pineal glands produce melatonin, which is vital for regulating cortisol, hormones, and body temperature. Even small amounts of artificial light can interrupt this process, suppressing melatonin (which is particularly sensitive to blue light), and this partially explains why so many of us have disrupted cortisol patterns. The stress hormone cortisol is supposed to be suppressed during sleep, but it's not in the presence of ambient light.

- So even a little bit of light in your bedroom at night, especially blue light, can disrupt hormones and potentially lead to weight gain, blood sugar problems, increased cancer risk, higher chance of depression and anxiety, premature aging, and heart problems. Fortunately, there are some easy solutions you can try: Get your bedroom (and your child's bedroom) as dark as possible by covering light sources and removing any unnecessary electronics.

- Install f.lux software (it's free) on all computers and devices to reduce blue light and help you sleep better (it's also easier on the eyes!).

- If you have artificial light outside (like streetlights), use blackout curtains to cover your windows.

- Avoid computers, phone screens, and TV for at least ninety minutes prior to bedtime. If you must use them, wear orange-tinted glasses to block blue spectrum light.

Keep Your Cool

Temperature is another important factor for great sleep. Your body temperature naturally cools slightly during sleep, and this occurs most easily when your bedroom is at certain temperatures. Temperature makes such a difference, in fact, that one initial study showed that insomniacs who wore cooling caps that helped reduce body temperature were able to sleep as soundly and for the same amount of time as those without any sleep disorders or problems. Most health experts recommend a bedroom temperature between 62°F and 68°F.

STAGING SLEEP

Not all sleep is created equal. There are several stages of sleep that the body cycles through during the night:

- N1: This is the stage during which you feel half-asleep and still have some awareness of your surroundings. This is also the stage where you involuntarily jerk or kick.

- N2: This is a slightly deeper stage of sleep. You actually spend about half of your sleeping hours in this stage.

- N3: This is the deep, slow sleep stage, in which your core temperature drops and your melatonin production increases. N3 cycles put you into the most "productive" of the sleep cycles.

- REM: Rapid eye movement sleep is when most dreaming occurs. In REM sleep, your muscles completely relax, and your mind and body regenerate at an amazing rate. Although only about a quarter of your daily sleep is REM, it is vitally important to healing and restoration.

There is also a technique called cold therapy for improving sleep. Popularized by Dr. Jack Kruse, this method has been around for a while, and if done correctly, it can help you sleep like a rock—and perhaps help with a host of problems such as chronic fatigue, heart issues, and possibly cancer and tumors.

From what I've read about cold therapy, full immersion in a cool bath (below 60°F) is most effective, although placing a cold ice pack on the front and back of your neck (as suggested by best-selling author Tim Ferriss) can help enhance sleep and weight loss. I'm still working up to full-body immersion (which I dread), but I've noticed a difference in my sleeping patterns from using cold therapy in one of these two ways:

- Sitting with ice packs on the front and back of my neck for thirty minutes

- Dipping my face in a bowl of very cold water (about 50°F) and holding it underwater for as long as I can, up to thirty seconds. I do this several times, and it definitely helps reduce stress and improve sleep. There is a theory that this activates the dive reflex, which helps reduce stress.

As for temperature and sleep quality, here's what I suggest:

- Keep your bedroom at a cool but comfortable temperature for you.

- Choose bedding that warms but doesn't make you hot.

- Place an ice pack on your forehead or on the back of your neck.

- Try cold therapy, from the ice packs to full immersion.

Play All the Right Noise

Many people use sound machines that generate white noise to block out intrusive racket. The low whir of a fan or an air conditioner does the same. But there's a caveat: Some studies suggest that these artificial forms of white noise can create a cortisol response in the body and that over the long term they may even impair brain function and development in children.

For years, we'd let our children fall asleep listening to choral music, soothing classical, or even Gregorian chants. But after they broke about six CD players, and we realized that CDs and CD players are getting harder to buy, we needed a better solution. We bought these two options:

Sleep Genius App. It provides soothing ambient noise without the high-pitched white noise frequencies found in most sound machines and other apps. At only $5, this app provides the correct frequencies of ambient noise. It won't raise cortisol or impair mental function and that helps the brain sleep more restfully. I use this in our bedroom but also turn my phone on airplane mode at night (to avoid call/text interruptions and the Wi-Fi and cell tower signal).

Wholetones Sleep System. Wholetones, through CDs or mini-speakers, plays frequency-based music that is designed to support the brain, body, and sleep. The idea is that certain frequencies of music have a soothing effect on the body. Find it here: WellnessMama.com/go/wholetones.

Invest in a Good Mattress

I feel like our mattress-seeking saga could be a book on its own. For years, we slept on a brand-new mattress that we bought for $100 on Craigslist. It worked and was comfortable. It wasn't a natural mattress, however, and it started to really show its wear after about seven years (helped along by a bunch of toddlers bouncing on it while I folded laundry).

After trying three natural mattress companies, we finally found a mattress that is both nontoxic and comfortable. Look for a mattress that is GOTS certified (the Global Organic Textile Standard for textiles like cotton and wool) or GOLS certified (the Global Organic Latex Standard for natural latex) and that doesn't contain added flame retardants.

UP YOUR AIR QUALITY

Air quality can directly affect sleep. The Harvard School of Public Health found that poor indoor air quality increased the risk of sleep disorders, including sleep apnea, which is one of the fastest growing sleep disorders. Indoor air pollution and the resulting sleep disorders may also increase the risk of cardiovascular disease.

This makes sense because we are sedentary and indoors at night, and are breathing more indoor air, which we know is often up to seventy times more polluted than outdoor air.

DIET YOUR WAY TO QUALITY SLEEP

To get that perfect night's sleep, change some of your daylight activities, including what you eat. Just as foods can impact health in other areas, foods can contribute to good or bad sleep. Here are some of the best foods to consume:

- **Healthful Fats.** These include my faves: coconut oil, organic and pasture-raised meats, eggs, avocados, and butter. They provide your body with the necessary building blocks to manufacture sleep hormones.

- **Foods High in Antioxidants.** These are important for hormone production and removal of toxins that can impede sleep. Focus on vegetables, nutrient-dense fruits (pomegranates, blueberries, cherries, grapes), and herbal or green teas (green tea early in the day only, because of the caffeine).

- **Quality Proteins.** Eating enough protein, especially at dinner, will help prepare the body to enter the sleep cycle. Stop eating at least four hours before bedtime, preferably by 6 p.m. every night. Your evening meal should include proteins, vegetables, and healthful fats.

Unfortunately, there are foods and substances that will have you tossing and turning all night, so avoid these if possible:

- **Grains.** I'm always on the soapbox about the negative effects grains can have on the body. If you're highly intolerant of grains, this can cause physical stress in your body, which alters the hormone cycle and can impede sleep.

- **Caffeine.** Depending on how sensitive you are to caffeine, even small amounts early in the day can inhibit sleep. Most caffeine-containing drinks and foods are bad for you anyway, so get rid of them. Especially avoid caffeine after noon.

- **Alcohol.** A glass of wine is a common way to wind down in the evening. Even though alcohol can cause drowsiness, it can prevent the body from entering the deeper and more regenerative sleep stages.

4-7-8 . . . BREATHE!

My massage therapist recommended this method to me; she learned it from the noted physician and celebrated author Dr. Andrew Weil. It involves a slow and patterned breathing that helps oxygenate the blood and promote relaxation.

When I researched this type of breathing, I learned that many religions use some variation of it for meditation or prayer. Recent information suggests that it may help the body shift from sympathetic nervous activity (fight or flight) to parasympathetic (relaxation) activity. Either way, it is a quick and simple technique that seems to really help promote restful sleep, and it doesn't cost a thing.

Here's how to do it:

Sit in a relaxed position or lie down. Breathe in through your nose as you count to four.

Hold your breath as you count to seven.

Slowly exhale through your mouth as you count to eight.

Repeat this pattern three or four times, or until you feel relaxed.

PUT YOUR FEET UP—THE RIGHT WAY

I picked up this sleep-well tip from a friend who had reversed his own health struggles through diet and lifestyle changes. Many of us are standing, walking, or (hopefully not) sitting for most of the day. As a result, blood and lymph fluid can collect in the legs. This is often more noticeable during pregnancy or if there is an underlying medical condition. If you've had kids, did you notice your feet and ankles being slightly more tired/sore/swollen at night when you were pregnant?

The simple and free solution is to elevate your feet for fifteen to thirty minutes at night. The ways that seem to be most effective are lying on the floor and resting the feet on a couch or chair at a 90-degree angle or lying on the floor or bed and resting the legs straight up against the wall (which is a little more difficult).

I try to do this every night because it helps me sleep so much better. Some nights, we do this as a family while we read books or do our family nighttime routine. Sound boring? Try reading or listening to a podcast while elevating your legs.

Here's my "overachiever version": If you want the benefits of elevating your feet along with the benefits of inversion, consider trying an inversion table or gravity boots. There is some evidence that full inversion can help joints and might help alleviate back pain. Both of these options let you essentially hang upside down and help stretch muscles and joints.

TRY NATURAL SLEEP REMEDIES

Some of the same remedies I've recommended previously for good health will also help provide a better night's sleep, namely cod liver oil, coconut oil, magnesium, and gelatin.

But here are some additional remedies you might want to consider for quality sleep:

- **Chamomile Tea.** I often drink a cup of chamomile or other herbal tea with a tablespoon of gelatin dissolved in it each night a couple hours prior to bedtime. Catnip tea works well too. The heat of a warm cup of tea will temporarily raise body temperature slightly, and the resulting drop will help you sleep.

- **Tart Cherry Juice.** This unusual remedy comes highly recommended in online reviews but has some scientific backing as well. Studies show that it may help with insomnia, improve melatonin levels, and reduce inflammation to promote restful sleep. It may even help improve how long we sleep. Case in point: Researchers from Louisiana State University had seven older adults with insomnia drink eight ounces of the juice twice a day for two weeks, followed by two weeks of no juice, and then two more weeks of drinking a placebo beverage. Compared with the placebo, drinking the cherry juice resulted in an average of eighty-four more minutes of sleep time each night.

  I drink a tablespoon of tart cherry juice at night to help with my own sleep quality, especially on days with intense workouts, because the juice also seems to help with muscle recovery and stiffness. Cherry juice can even be added to chamomile tea or other relaxing herbal teas (with the honey salt remedy on page 129) to help improve the taste.

- **Homemade Sleep Tincture.** My sleep tinctures are among my favorite sleep remedies, made from some of my favorite herbs. We don't have to use them often, but when one of the kids is sick, or we are traveling and the kids are off-schedule, this natural tincture helps them sleep peacefully. See Chapter 19 for all my homemade sleep remedies.

MAINTAIN A CONSISTENT DAILY ROUTINE

Staying on a consistent routine each day helps ensure the greatest amount of quality sleep. This is because your circadian rhythm, the internal time-keeping clock for the body, remains constant, and your hormone production is optimal. The most beneficial hours of sleep are between 10 p.m. and 2 a.m., though most adults miss about half of this. It seems that we are good at holding our kids to a strict sleep schedule, but as often is the case, this is a "do as I say, not as I do" situation.

A daily (and nightly) routine can make a big difference in how easily you fall and stay asleep. You'll have to experiment to find out what works best for you, but here are some helpful suggestions for daily consistency:

- Wake up and go to bed at the same time, even on weekends, to keep your hormone cycle regular. In fact, try to get to bed by 10 p.m. This will ensure the greatest amount of quality sleep. Your adrenals recharge your body during these hours, and it releases more bile (a backup of this can lead to gallbladder stones).

- Eat a high-protein, high-fat snack a few hours before bed (7 p.m. or earlier) or consume a lot at dinner.

- Stay hydrated during the day, but stop drinking water and other fluids a couple hours before bedtime to prevent interrupting sleep with trips to the bathroom.

- Take a soothing warm bath about an hour before bedtime.

- Get at least a half hour of sunlight each day (even if you aren't trying to get your vitamin D). Adequate exposure to daylight elevates levels of feel-good serotonin, a neurotransmitter that helps improve sleep-inducing melatonin levels at night.

- Pray, meditate, or find another way to reduce stress.

- Stretch before bed to relax muscles.

- Trade out your jolting, buzzing alarm clock for a gentle sunlight alarm clock that will wake you up much more gently. I don't know about you, but my dread of the sound of the alarm clock sound always causes me to wake up a few times in the early morning in anticipation of it.

- Try an earthing mat. I am still experimenting with this one, but there is some evidence that sleeping on an earthing mat reduces your exposure to low-frequency electromagnetic fields and improves sleep quality. While I have noticed a big difference on myself, I don't know how much of this effect is psychological, so I'm experimenting with having the kids sleep on it without them knowing what it does. The book *Earthing* explains more of the theory behind this method, and I'm working on finding a good source of the mats. According to the book, you can also create the same effect by spending time barefoot outside on dirt, grass, or rocks daily for at least a half hour. (If you garden barefoot in the middle of the day, you'll get three benefits in one—from exercise, vitamin D, and the negative electrons from the earth.)

- Exercise (just not right before bed!). Besides the plethora of other benefits of daily exercise, exercising during the day can help the body function optimally so that sleep hormone production is optimal.

I hope that these tips will be as helpful to you as they are to my family. Certainly, not every option will fit every budget, but even creating a no-cost darker, cooler sleep environment can help you reap the benefits of a more restful night's sleep.

the recipes

···

Note: All of the ingredients for these recipes can be found at WellnessMama.com/detox-book/

wellness mama life detox recipes

I've always loved to cook, experiment with new dishes, and basically just tinker around in the kitchen. As I followed my heart to pursue healthful living, I realized that I could make my own natural remedies, beauty products, and cleaning solutions at home—and it was such a freeing, empowering experience. Best of all, it's easy!

As for natural remedies, there is still a time and a place for traditional medicine, of course, but for minor illnesses and ailments, it is great to have home remedies to turn to. It took me years to develop and incorporate all of these recipes, so don't feel like you have to jump into all of them at once! I recommend starting with a few simple but really effective remedies— elderberry syrup, herbal teas, and a salve or two—and build from there.

You will love concocting your own beauty products. We all want beautiful skin, and as you now know, much of skin health comes from the inside out. We can also naturally support skin without slathering on dozens of questionable chemicals using a few natural items. The fun part of natural beauty recipes is the experimentation! You get to figure out exactly what works for your skin type and customize to your exact specifications. I'd suggest starting with basic oil cleaning and a simple sugar scrub. From there, branch out into more complicated recipes like makeup and lotions.

Cleaning products are probably the easiest of all, because they require so few ingredients. Best of all, you won't be exposing yourself or your family to harmful chemicals. Once you get on board with natural cleaning products, you'll be detoxing right away.

As you can see, detoxing your life provides so many amazing benefits. It's just a matter of starting with a few recipes and progressing from there. Just have fun and you'll begin to look forward to creating health magic right in your own kitchen. These recipes are meant to empower you to create incredibly healthful alternatives that will give you and your family better health for years to come.

If you don't have all of these ingredients on hand already, check out the easy reference sheet of where to find them at WellnessMama.com/detox-book/.

Natural Medicine Recipes

Elderberry Syrup

⅔ cup dried black elderberries

2 tablespoons minced peeled fresh ginger or ground ginger

1 teaspoon ground cinnamon

½ teaspoon whole or ground cloves

1 cup raw honey (we get ours at our farmers' market)

In a medium saucepan, bring to a boil 3½ cups water. Add the elderberries, ginger, cinnamon, and cloves, then reduce the heat, cover, and simmer until the liquid is reduced by almost half, 45 minutes to 1 hour. Remove from the heat and let cool enough to be handled.

Mash the berries carefully with a spoon or other flat utensil.

Pour through a strainer into a clean pint-size mason jar. Discard the solids and let the liquid cool to lukewarm. Add the honey and stir well. Cap tightly and store in the refrigerator for up to two weeks.

For adults, take ½ to 1 tablespoon daily for its immune-boosting properties. For children, take ½ to 1 teaspoon daily. Some sources recommend taking only during the week and not on the weekends to boost immunity because the body can adapt if taken every day so it's more effective when intake is on a cycle. If the flu does strike, take the normal dose every 2 to 3 hours, instead of once a day, until symptoms disappear.

NOTE: For children under two years old, maple syrup may be used instead of honey. If avoiding all sweeteners, this can be consumed without a sweetener or a few drops of stevia can be added to the finished mixture instead of honey. Please note that the mixture will not last as long if honey is not used, as it works as a natural preservative.

Lemon-Cinnamon Cough Syrup

1 quart filtered water

¼ cup minced peeled fresh ginger

¼ cup dried chamomile flowers

¼ cup dried marshmallow root

1 tablespoon ground cinnamon

¼ cup lemon juice

1 cup honey

In a medium saucepan, bring the water to a boil. Add the ginger, flowers, marshmallow root powder, and cinnamon. Reduce the heat and simmer uncovered for 15 to 20 minutes, until reduced by at least half and the herbs have infused into water. Remove from the heat and let cool slightly.

Pour through a strainer into a clean quart-size mason jar. Discard the solids. When the liquid has cooled slightly but is still warm, add the lemon juice and honey and stir well. Cap tightly and store in the refrigerator for up to 2 weeks.

Herbal Throat Spray

This herbal throat spray eases the pain of a sore throat. It has a double benefit as it is an herbal syrup combined with a tincture. This throat spray is essentially a strong herbal tincture mixed with raw honey. The herbs provide both immediate relief and longer-lasting benefits for beating illness.

1 tablespoon dried echinacea root
1 tablespoon ground ginger
1 tablespoon dried marshmallow root
1 tablespoon dried elderberries
1 tablespoon dried thyme
1 tablespoon dried mint
$\frac{1}{2}$ teaspoon ground cayenne pepper
1 cup food-grade alcohol, such as rum or vodka
$\frac{1}{4}$ cup raw honey

Place the echinacea root, ginger, marshmallow root, elderberries, thyme, mint, and cayenne in a pint-size jar and cover with the alcohol. Cap tightly and let rest for 6 to 8 weeks, shaking daily.

Pour through a strainer into a clean pint-size mason jar. Discard the solids. Pour the tincture into a pint size or larger mason jar and store in a cool dry place for up to 2 years. This mixture is very shelf stable and will last that long until mixed with honey. Once you add the honey (see next step), it should only be stored for up to 3 weeks in the fridge.

To use, mix 3 tablespoons of the tincture with 1 tablespoon honey and shake or stir until combined. Store the mixture in a small spray bottle and use as needed as a throat spray for sore throat.

Variation: If you prefer not to make a tincture with alcohol, you can make a vegetable glycerine tincture instead or just use a strong tea and mix with honey. If you want to use the full herbal mixture and don't have weeks to sit around for the tincture, you can make a 2-hour tincture with this method:
Combine 1 teaspoon of all of the herbs you want to use in a small glass jar. Pour over enough boiling water to just cover the herbs. Let steep for 20 minutes and let cool. Strain out the solids and mix with equal parts alcohol (I use rum or vodka). Use this mixture to make the spray as usual.

Spicy Cider Immune Boost

I first discovered a recipe for "fire cider" a few years ago when I got a copy of Rosemary Gladstar's *Medicinal Herbs* book, which shares this recipe and many others. It is a traditional recipe that contains garlic, onion, ginger, cayenne, vinegar, and raw honey. Her recipe also calls for horseradish, but I typically substitute echinacea root. Judging by the ingredients in the recipe, you might not expect it to taste very good. I didn't either, but I was quite pleasantly surprised by the taste. I've even tried it on salads as a dressing and it has a mild peppery and sweet vinaigrette flavor. I like to mix with more honey for a syrup (see next recipe).

In the winter months, I sometimes take a teaspoon or so of this a day or use it on salads. If illness hits, I'll take that dose every few hours or add a tablespoon to hot water or herbal tea a few times a day until I feel better.

1 medium onion, roughly chopped

1 head of garlic, cloves separated and roughly chopped

2 tablespoons grated peeled fresh ginger

1 tablespoon dried echinacea root (optional)

2 teaspoons ground cayenne pepper

Apple cider vinegar (organic and with the "mother"), such as Bragg

Place the onion, garlic, ginger, echinacea root (if using), and cayenne pepper in a quart-size mason jar. Add enough vinegar just to cover. Cap tightly and let rest in a sunny, warm (not hot) place for 2 to 3 weeks.

Pour through a strainer into a clean quart-size mason jar. Discard the solids. Cap tightly and store in the refrigerator or a cool, dark place for up to 1 year.

To use, take 1 teaspoon as needed daily or when illness strikes. I've taken as much as 1 teaspoon an hour during illness until I felt better.

Spicy Cider Syrup

½ cup Spicy Cider Immune Boost (page 127)
½ cup raw honey

In a pint-size mason jar, mix together the cider immune boost and honey and stir to combine. Cap tightly and store in refrigerator for up to 2 weeks. Consume as needed.

Cinnamon Honey for Cold Relief

½ cup raw honey
3 tablespoons ground cinnamon

In an 8-ounce mason jar, mix together the cinnamon and honey. Cap tightly and store for up to 1 year. Use as needed for immune support.

Rose-Infused Honey

½ cup raw honey
¼ cup dried organic rose petals

In an 8-ounce or larger mason jar, mix together the rose petals and honey. Cap tightly and let rest for at least 1 week to infuse. Strain out the petals, if desired, though I prefer to leave the petals in the honey for presentation and additional flavor. Store at room temperature for up to 2 years (though honey is one of the few substances that will never go bad). Makes a great gift.

Lavender Honey for Cuts, Burns, and Immune Health

½ cup raw honey

¼ cup dried lavender flowers (see Note)

In an 8-ounce or larger mason jar, mix together the honey and flowers. Cap tightly and let rest for 2 weeks to infuse. Strain out the flowers, if desired, or leave in the honey. Use as needed as a salve on cuts and burns. It may also be added to teas or drizzled on food for immune support.

Note: Alternatively, you can use 15 drops food-grade lavender essential oil in place of the dried lavender. If you do this, there is no need to wait 2 weeks to let it infuse.

Chamomile Honey Salt for Bedtime

My kids call this "honey salt" and ask for it some nights. The combination of sweet and salty in a small amount can help promote restful sleep.

½ cup raw honey

¼ cup dried chamomile flowers

1 tablespoon salt

In an 8-ounce or larger mason jar, mix together the honey and flowers. Cap tightly and let rest for at least 4 weeks to infuse.

Pour through a strainer into a clean 8-ounce mason jar. Discard the solids. Add the salt and mix well. Cap tightly and store at room temperature for up to a year.

To use, take 1 tablespoon at night before bed.

Marshmallow-Mint Sore Throat Honey

½ cup raw honey
2 tablespoons dried marshmallow root
2 tablespoons dried peppermint

In an 8-ounce or larger mason jar, mix together the honey, marshmallow root, and peppermint. Cap tightly and let rest for at least 4 weeks to infuse. Strain out the herbs, if desired, or leave in the honey.

To use, take 1 teaspoon as needed either alone or added to an herbal tea for sore throat relief.

Vanilla Honey for Tea

½ cup raw honey
3 whole vanilla beans

Pour the honey in an 8-ounce or larger mason jar. Slice the vanilla beans lengthwise and scrape out and discard the seeds. Cut the pods into 1-inch pieces and add to the honey. Cap tightly and let rest for 3 to 4 weeks to infuse.

To use, stir a teaspoon into a cup of your favorite tea.

Thyme Honey for Cough

½ cup raw honey
¼ cup dried thyme

In an 8-ounce or larger mason jar, mix together the honey and thyme. Cap tightly and let rest for at least 4 weeks to infuse. Strain if desired. Store in a cool, dark place for up to a year.

To use, take 1 teaspoon of the mixture as needed to soothe cough.

Sleep Easy Tea Blend

My go-to tea when I am having trouble sleeping is an equal mixture of chamomile, mint, and catnip. Use the same mixture to fill a homemade eye pillow to aid in sleep as well.

    1 tablespoon dried chamomile flowers
    1 tablespoon dried mint
    1 teaspoon dried catnip (optional)

In a small glass jar, mix together the flowers, mint, and (if using) the catnip. Cap tightly and store in the pantry for up to 6 months.

To use, add 1 to 2 teaspoons per cup of water to make hot or iced tea.

Lavender Tea

Lavender is my favorite scent and essential oil, but it is too strong to be used alone in a tea. Here is my solution for a relaxing tea.

    ½ cup dried mint
    2 tablespoons dried lavender flowers
    2 tablespoons dried stevia leaf (optional)

In a small glass jar, mix together the mint, flowers, and (if using) the stevia. Cap tightly and store in the pantry for up to 6 months.

To use, add 1 to 2 teaspoons per cup of water to make hot or iced tea.

Stomach Soother Tea

For stomachaches or other mild digestive troubles, this tea is very calming.

 2 teaspoons dried mint
 ½ teaspoon fennel seeds
 Pinch of ground ginger (optional)
 1 cup boiling water

Place the mint, fennel seeds, and (if using) the ginger in a mug. Pour in the boiling water, cover, and steep for 5 minutes. For a long-lasting soothing effect, you can also add 1 tablespoon gelatin powder.

Happy Hormone Tea

Red raspberry is known to be great for hormone balance and women's health. The mint and nettle add a variety of other nutrients, and stevia adds a hint of sweetness.

 4 cups dried red raspberry leaf
 ½ cup dried mint
 ¼ cup dried stevia leaf, or to taste
 1 cup dried nettle leaf

In a 64-ounce mason jar, mix together all the ingredients. Cap tightly and store in the pantry for up to a year.

To use, add 1 tablespoon to brew by the mugful or 1 cup to brew by the gallon. Enjoy!

Immune-Boosting Turmeric Tea

Turmeric is getting a lot of press lately for its anti-inflammatory properties. Bodies absorb turmeric better when black pepper has been added to it. Many people love this ancient spice for its taste and health.

   2 cups coconut milk
   1 teaspoon ground turmeric
   1 teaspoon ground cinnamon
   1 teaspoon raw honey or pure maple syrup, or to taste
   Pinch of black pepper
   1-inch piece peeled fresh ginger or $\frac{1}{4}$ teaspoon ground ginger
   Pinch of cayenne pepper (optional)

Place the coconut milk, turmeric, cinnamon, honey, pepper, ginger, and (if using) the cayenne in a high-speed blender and blend until smooth.

Pour into a small saucepan over medium heat. Divide between two mugs.

Immune-Boosting Elderberry Tea

Elderberries are delicious and are known in folk remedies for their immune-boosting properties. I love them for their taste and many health benefits, and this tea is a staple in our home, especially during the winter.

16 ounces filtered water

2 tablespoons dried elderberries

1/2 teaspoon ground turmeric

1/4 teaspoon ground cinnamon

1 teaspoon raw honey (optional)

In a small saucepan, bring to a boil the water, elderberries, turmeric, and cinnamon. Reduce the heat and simmer for about 15 minutes to extract the beneficial properties of the elderberries. Remove from the heat and let cool for about 5 minutes.

Pour through a strainer into a pint-size mason jar, then discard the solids. Divide the tea between two mugs. Stir in the honey (if using).

For iced tea, leave in the mason jar and stir in honey (if desired). Let cool, then refrigerate until cold.

Arnica Oil for Bruises and Soreness

(External Use Only on Unbroken Skin)

 ½ cup dried arnica flowers
 1 cup olive, almond, or other carrier oil

Place the flowers in a pint-size mason jar. Cover with oil, leaving at least 1 inch oil above the flowers and 1 inch at top of jar. Cap tightly and let rest in a cool, dark place for 4 to 6 weeks, shaking every few days. Strain out as needed for homemade lotions and salves.

Calendula Oil for Healthy Skin (External Use Only)

 ½ cup calendula flowers
 1 cup olive, almond, or other carrier oil

Place the flowers in a pint-size mason jar. Cover with oil, leaving at least 1 inch oil above the flowers and 1 inch at top of jar. Cap tightly and let rest in a cool, dark place for 4 to 6 weeks, shaking every few days. Strain out as needed for homemade lotions and salves.

St. John's Wort Oil for Bruises and Skin Irritation
(External Use Only)

½ cup St. John's wort flowers
1 cup olive, almond, or other carrier oil

Place the flowers in a pint-size mason jar. Cover with oil, leaving at least 1 inch oil above the herb and 1 inch at top of jar. Cap tightly and let rest in a cool, dark place for 4 to 6 weeks, shaking every few days. Strain out as needed for homemade lotions and salves.

Myrrh Gum Oil for Skin Infections (External Use Only)

2 tablespoons myrrh gum
½ cup olive, almond, or other carrier oil

Place the myrrh gum in a pint-size mason jar. Cover with oil, leaving at least 1 inch oil above the gum and 1 inch at top of jar. Cap tightly and let rest in a cool, dark place for 4 to 6 weeks, shaking every few days. Strain out as needed for homemade lotions and salves.

Plantain Oil for Cuts, Scrapes, and Bites

(External Use Only)

Plantain is another backyard herb with a lot of benefits. It always grows near poison ivy and other harmful plants, and it is a natural remedy for itching, bug bites, and more. I've taught my children what it looks like and how to find a leaf and use it on bee stings and mosquito bites to reduce the pain or itch. It is also great in poultices like this and can be used for all types of skin problems.

$\frac{1}{2}$ cup dried plantain leaf
1 cup olive, almond, or other carrier oil

Place the plantain leaf in a pint-size mason jar. Cover with oil, leaving at least 1 inch of oil above the herb and 1 inch at top of jar. Cap tightly and let rest in a cool, dark place for 4 to 6 weeks, shaking every few days. Strain out as needed for homemade lotions and salves.

Rosemary Oil for Scalp Health and Hair Growth

(External Use Only)

$\frac{1}{2}$ cup dried rosemary
1 cup olive, almond, or other carrier oil

Place rosemary in a pint-size mason jar. Cover with oil, leaving at least 1 inch of oil above the herb and 1 inch at top of jar. Cap tightly and let rest in a cool, dark place for 4 to 6 weeks, shaking every few days. Strain out as needed for homemade hair treatments.

These salves use herb-infused oils as the base.

Substitutions: Reduce beeswax to ¼ cup and add 2 tablespoons of shea butter. If you use coconut oil to infuse the oils, you will also reduce the beeswax to ¼ cup, even if not using shea butter.

Echinacea and Goldenseal Antibiotic Salve (External Use Only)

1 cup echinacea flower and goldenseal infused oil (see page 50)
⅓ cup beeswax pastilles
4 drops tea tree essential oil (optional)

In a double boiler over low heat, completely melt the infused oil and beeswax. Remove from the heat and add the essential oil (if using). Quickly pour into small tins or jars and let cool and harden completely. Cap tightly and store at room temperature for up to 3 years. (At temperatures above 85°F, the salve will melt.) Use as needed on affected skin.

Black Walnut Salve for Fungus and Ringworm
(External Use Only)

1 cup black walnut powder infused oil (see page 50)

⅓ cup beeswax pastilles

5 drops tea tree essential oil (optional)

2 drops oregano essential oil (optional)

In a double boiler over low heat, completely melt the infused oil and beeswax. Remove from the heat and add the essential oil (if using). Quickly pour into small tins or jars and let cool and harden completely. Cap tightly and store at room temperature for up to 3 years. (At temperatures above 85°F, the salve will melt.) Use as needed on affected skin.

Sleepytime Salve (External Use Only)

1 cup chamomile flower, valerian root, and catnip infused oil (see page 50)

⅓ cup beeswax pastilles

15 drops lavender essential oil (optional)

In a double boiler over low heat, completely melt the infused oil and beeswax. Remove from the heat and add the essential oil (if using). Quickly pour into small tins or jars and let cool and harden completely. (At temperatures above 85°F, the salve will melt.) Use as needed on skin.

Breathe Easy Salve (External Use Only)

1 cup eucalyptus-infused oil (see page 50)

⅓ cup beeswax pastilles

3 drops peppermint essential oil

3 drops eucalyptus essential oil

In a double boiler over low heat, completely melt the infused oil and beeswax. Remove from the heat and add the essential oil (if using). Quickly pour into small tins or jars and let cool and harden completely. Cap tightly and store at room temperature for up to 3 years. (At temperatures above 85°F, the salve will melt.) For adult use only. Apply to feet or chest as needed.

Menthol Peppermint Salve for Sore Muscles (External Use Only)

1 cup peppermint leaf (⅓ cup) and menthol crystal (optional 1 teaspoon) infused oil (see page 50)

⅓ cup beeswax pastilles

10 drops peppermint essential oil

In a double boiler over low heat, completely melt the infused oil and beeswax. Remove from the heat and add the essential oil (if using). Quickly pour into small tins or jars and let cool and harden completely. Cap tightly and store at room temperature for up to 3 years. (At temperatures above 85°F, the salve will melt.) Use as needed on tired, sore muscles. For adult use only.

Peppermint Headache Salve (External Use Only)

1 cup peppermint-infused oil (see page 50)

⅓ cup beeswax pastilles

10 drops peppermint essential oil

3 drops wintergreen essential oil (optional)

In a double boiler over low heat, completely melt the infused oil and beeswax. Remove from the heat and add the essential oil (if using). Quickly pour into small tins or jars and let cool and harden completely. Cap tightly and store at room temperature for up to 3 years. (At temperatures above 85°F, the salve will melt.) Use on neck and head as needed, being careful to avoid the eyes. Adult use only.

Burn and Blister Salve (External Use Only)

1 cup plantain leaf and lavender infused oil (see page 50)

⅓ cup beeswax pastilles

20 drops lavender essential oil (optional)

In a double boiler over low heat, completely melt the infused oil and beeswax. Remove from the heat and add the essential oil (if using). Quickly pour into small tins or jars and let cool and harden completely. Cap tightly and store at room temperature for up to 3 years. (At temperatures above 85°F, the salve will melt.) Use as needed on affected skin.

Note: This should not be applied immediately after a burn. Allow heat to escape first. For immediate application, instead use Lavender Honey for Cuts, Burns, and Immune Health (page 129). Always seek medical help immediately for severe burns.

Chamomile Calming Balm (External Use Only)

1 cup chamomile-infused oil (see page 50)

⅓ cup beeswax pastilles

5 drops lavender essential oil (optional)

5 drops chamomile essential oil (optional)

In a double boiler over low heat, completely melt the infused oil and beeswax. Remove from the heat and add the essential oils (if using). Quickly pour into small tins or jars and let cool and harden completely. Cap tightly and store at room temperature for up to 3 years. (At temperatures above 85°F, the salve will melt.) Use as needed on skin—this is especially good for rubbing on children's feet before bed to improve sleep.

Plantain Salve for Skin Healing (External Use Only)

1 cup plantain oil (see page 137)

⅓ cup beeswax pastilles

20 drops lavender essential oil (optional)

10 drops frankincense essential oil (optional)

In a double boiler over low heat, completely melt the infused oil and beeswax. Remove from the heat and add the essential oils (if using). Quickly pour into small tins or jars and let cool and harden completely. Cap tightly and store at room temperature for up to 3 years. (At temperatures above 85°F, the salve will melt.) Use as needed on skin.

Lavender Smooth Skin Salve (External Use Only)

1 cup lavender and calendula infused oil (see page 50)
⅓ cup beeswax pastilles
30 drops lavender essential oil (optional)
10 drops patchouli essential oil (optional)

In a double boiler over low heat, completely melt the infused oil and beeswax. Remove from the heat and add the essential oils (if using). Quickly pour into small tins or jars and let cool and harden completely. Cap tightly and store at room temperature for up to 3 years. (At temperatures above 85°F, the salve will melt.) Use as needed on skin.

Antiaging Salve (External Use Only)

1 cup lavender, calendula, and rose infused oil (see page 50)
⅓ cup beeswax pastilles
10 drops rose essential oil (optional)

In a double boiler over low heat, completely melt the infused oil and beeswax. Remove from the heat and add the essential oil (if using). Quickly pour into small tins or jars and let cool and harden completely. Cap tightly and store at room temperature for up to 3 years. (At temperatures above 85°F, the salve will melt.) Use as needed on skin.

Hormone Balance Salve (External Use Only)

1 cup red raspberry leaf and clary sage infused oil (see page 50)

⅓ cup beeswax pastilles

10 drops lavender essential oil (optional)

5 drops clary sage essential oil (optional)

In a double boiler over low heat, completely melt the infused oil and beeswax. Remove from the heat and add the essential oils (if using). Quickly pour into small tins or jars and let cool and harden completely. Cap tightly and store at room temperature for up to 3 years. (At temperatures above 85°F, the salve will melt.) Use as needed on skin. Adult use only.

Garlic-Rosemary Antibacterial Salve (External Use Only)

1 cup raw garlic and rosemary infused oil (see page 50)

⅓ cup beeswax pastilles

5 drops rosemary essential oil (optional)

In a double boiler over low heat, completely melt the infused oil and beeswax. Remove from the heat and add rosemary essential oil (if using). Quickly pour into tins or jars and let cool and harden completely. Cap tightly and store at room temperature for up to 3 years. (At temperatures above 85°F, the salve will melt.) Use as needed on affected skin.

Achy Foot Salve (External Use Only)

1 cup peppermint and rosemary infused oil (see page 50)

⅓ cup beeswax pastilles

10 drops peppermint essential oil (optional)

In a double boiler over low heat, completely melt the infused oil and beeswax. Remove from the heat and add the essential oil (if using). Quickly pour into small tins or jars and let cool and harden completely. Cap tightly and store at room temperature for up to 3 years. (At temperatures above 85°F, the salve will melt.) Use as needed to soothe tired, achy feet.

Cracked Heel Salve (External Use Only)

peppermint (¼ cup) and cayenne (1 teaspoon) infused oil (see page 50)

¼ cup beeswax pastilles

2 tablespoons shea butter

10 drops rosemary essential oil (optional)

15 drops lavender essential oil (optional)

10 drops lemon essential oi (optional)

In a double boiler over low heat, completely melt the infused oil and beeswax. Remove from the heat and add the essential oils (if using). Quickly pour into small tins or jars and let cool and harden completely. Cap tightly and store at room temperature for up to 3 years. (At temperatures above 85°F, the salve will melt.) Use as needed to moisturize dry, cracked heels. Adult use only.

Anti-Itch Salve (External Use Only)

1 cup nettle, plantain, and rosemary infused oil (see page 50)

⅓ cup beeswax pastilles

½ teaspoon baking soda

25 drops lavender essential oil (optional)

In a double boiler over low heat, completely melt the infused oil and beeswax. Stir in the baking soda. Remove from the heat and add the essential oil (if using). Quickly pour into small tins or jars and let cool and harden completely. Cap tightly and store at room temperature for up to 3 years. (At temperatures above 85°F, the salve will melt.) Use as needed on affected skin.

Castor Oil Hair Growth Salve for Men (External Use Only)

1 cup nettle-infused castor oil (see page 50)

2 tablespoons beeswax pastilles

8 drops rosemary essential oil (optional)

In a double boiler over low heat, completely melt the infused oil and beeswax. Remove from the heat and add the essential oil (if using). Quickly pour into small tins or jars and let cool and harden completely. Cap tightly and store at room temperature for up to 3 years. (At temperatures above 85°F, the salve will melt.)

This is best for men, as it is difficult to get out of longer hair. Massage a tiny amount into the scalp before bed. The infused castor oil can be used alone without the beeswax for great results as well. Adult use only.

Chickweed Soothing Salve (External Use Only)

1 cup chickweed-infused oil (see page 50)

1/3 cup beeswax pastilles

10 drops lavender essential oil (optional)

In a double boiler over low heat, completely melt the infused oil and beeswax. Remove from the heat and add the essential oil (if using). Quickly pour into small tins or jars and let cool and harden completely. Cap tightly and store at room temperature for up to 3 years. (At temperatures above 85°F, the salve will melt.) Use as needed on skin.

Emu Oil Intensive Skin Repair Salve (External Use Only)

1/4 cup emu oil

2 tablespoons shea butter

1 teaspoon beeswax pastilles

25 drops lavender essential oil (optional)

5 drops rosemary essential oil (optional)

In a double boiler, completely melt the emu oil, shea butter, and beeswax. Remove from the heat and add the essential oils (if using). Quickly pour into small tins or jars and let cool and harden completely. Cap tightly and store at room temperature for up to 3 years. (At temperatures above 85°F, the salve will melt.) Use as needed on skin. Adult use only if rosemary essential oil is added.

Pink Grapefruit Cellulite Salve (External Use Only)

1 cup rosemary and calendula infused oil (see page 50)

⅓ cup beeswax pastilles

20 drops pink grapefruit essential oil (optional)

In a double boiler over low heat, completely melt the infused oil and beeswax. Remove from the heat and add the essential oil (if using). Quickly pour into small tins or jars and let cool and harden completely. Cap tightly and store at room temperature for up to 3 years. (At temperatures above 85°F, the salve will melt.) Use as needed on cellulite. Adult use only.

Chamomile Tincture

$\frac{1}{2}$ to 1 cup dried chamomile flowers
Boiling water (about $\frac{1}{2}$ to $\frac{3}{4}$ cup)
$1\frac{1}{2}$ to $1\frac{3}{4}$ cups vodka or rum

Place the flowers in a quart-size mason jar and pour in just enough boiling water to cover (you may have to stir). Fill the rest of the jar with the vodka and cap tightly. Let rest in a cool, dark place for 4 to 6 weeks, shaking daily for the first 2 weeks. This will make a strong tincture!

Pour through a strainer into small glass jars or tincture vials. Discard the solids. Cap tightly and store in a cool, dark place for up to 2 years.

Calm Digestion Tincture

$\frac{1}{2}$ cup dried peppermint
$\frac{1}{4}$ to $\frac{1}{2}$ cup very finely diced peeled fresh ginger
$\frac{1}{4}$ cup fennel seeds
Boiling water
About $1\frac{1}{2}$ cups vodka or rum

Place the peppermint, ginger, and fennel seeds in a quart-size mason jar and pour in just enough boiling water to cover. Fill the rest of the jar with the vodka and cap tightly. Let rest in a cool, dark place for 2 to 6 weeks, shaking daily for the first 2 weeks.

Pour through a strainer into small glass jars or tincture vials. Discard the solids. Cap tightly and store in a cool, dark place for up to 2 years.

Soothe to Sleep Tincture

2 tablespoons dried yarrow flowers (relaxing and nutrient packed)

2 tablespoons dried catnip (naturally calming)

2 tablespoons dried oat straw (also helps with bed wetting)

2 tablespoons chamomile flowers (calming and relaxing)

1 tablespoon dried mint

1 tablespoon dried hops flowers

1 tablespoon dried stevia leaf

Boiling water

2 cups vodka or rum

Place all the flowers and herbs in a quart-size mason jar, pour in just enough boiling water to cover, and mix well. Fill the rest of the jar with the vodka and cap tightly. Let rest in a cool, dark place for 2 to 8 weeks, shaking daily for the first 2 weeks.

Pour through a strainer into small glass jars or tincture vials. Discard the solids. Cap tightly and store in a cool, dark place for up to 2 years.

For adults, take 2 to 3 dropperfuls. For children over age two, take 1 dropperful.

Plant-Based Multivitamin Tincture

3/4 cup dried alfalfa
1/2 cup dried red raspberry leaf
1/2 cup dried dandelion leaf
1/4 cup dried stevia leaf (optional; for taste)
1 cup boiling water
2 cups alcohol (vodka or rum)

Measurements are by volume (1 part = ¼ cup) or by weight (1 part = 1 ounce).

Fill a quart-size mason jar one-third to one-half full with all the ingredients. A half-full jar makes a stronger tincture. Do not pack down. Pour in the boiling water to just dampen. (This step is optional but helps to draw out the beneficial properties of the herbs.) Fill the rest of the jar with alcohol, give it a stir, and cap tightly. Let rest in a cool, dry place for at least 3 weeks and up to 6 months, shaking daily for the first 2 weeks (I usually leave herbs for 6 weeks).

Pour through a strainer into small glass jars or tincture vials. Cap tightly and store in a cool, dark place for up to 2 years.

White Willow Pain Relief Tincture

White willow was used as a source of salicylic acid to relieve pain before aspirin and pain relievers were invented. It is still often used for pain relief, especially joint pain.

1/2 cup dried white willow bark
Boiling water
1½ to 1¾ cups vodka or rum

Place the white willow in a quart-size mason jar and pour in just enough boiling water to cover (you may have to stir). Fill the rest of the jar with the vodka and cap tightly. Let rest in a cool, dark place for 4 to 6 weeks, shaking daily for the first 2 weeks. This will make a strong tincture!

Pour through a strainer into small glass jars or tincture vials. Discard the solids. Cap tightly and store in a cool, dark place for up to 2 years.

Valerian Insomnia-Busting Tincture

½ cup dried valerian root
Boiling water
1½ to 1¾ cups vodka or rum

Place the valerian in a quart-size mason jar and pour in just enough boiling water to cover (you may have to stir). Fill the rest of the jar with vodka and cap tightly. Let rest in a cool, dark place for 4 to 6 weeks, shaking daily for the first 2 weeks. This will make a strong tincture!

Pour through a strainer into small glass jars or tincture vials. Discard the solids. Cap tightly and store in a cool, dark place for up to 2 years.

Plantain Skin Tincture

Plantain is great for all types of skin troubles, and this tincture can be taken internally or applied externally on rashes, bites, and cuts and scrapes.

1 cup dried plantain leaf
Boiling water
1½ to 1¾ cups vodka or rum

Place the plantain leaf in a quart-size mason jar and pour in just enough boiling water to cover (you may have to stir). Fill the rest of the jar with vodka and cap tightly. Let rest in a cool, dark place for 4 to 6 weeks, shaking daily for the first 2 weeks. This will make a strong tincture!

Pour through a strainer into small glass jars or tincture vials. Discard the solids. Cap tightly and store in a cool, dark place for up to 2 years.

St. John's Wort Happy Tincture

St. John's wort is often recommended for anxiety and depression and its effects are cumulative. Many people see great results after using for at least a month. Of course, consult with a qualified professional before using this or any herb, especially for a mental health condition.

½ cup dried St. John's wort
Boiling water
1½ to 1¾ cups vodka or rum

Put the St. John's wort in a quart-size glass jar and pour in just enough boiling water to cover (you may have to stir). Fill the rest of the jar with vodka and cap tightly. Store in a cool, dark place for 4 to 6 weeks, shaking daily for the first 2 weeks. This will make a strong tincture!

Pour through a strainer into small glass jars or tincture vials. Discard the solids. Cap tightly and store in a cool, dark place for up to 2 years.

Dandelion Liver Boost Tincture

Many people think of dandelion as a pesky backyard weed. It also happens to be a potent and beneficial herb with a long history of use for supporting the liver and skin.

½ cup dried dandelion leaf
½ cup dried dandelion root
Boiling water
1½ to 1¾ cups vodka or rum

Place the dandelion leaf and root in a quart-size mason jar and pour in just enough boiling water to cover (you may have to stir). Fill the rest of the jar with vodka and cap tightly. Store in a cool, dark place for 4 to 6 weeks, shaking daily for the first 2 weeks. This will make a strong tincture!

Pour through a strainer into small glass jars or tincture vials. Discard the solids. Cap tightly and store in a cool, dark place for up to 2 years.

How to Make a Glycerite

Boiling water
Food-grade vegetable glycerine
Dried herbs of choice

Fill a pint-size mason jar one-third to one-half full with dried herbs. A half-full jar makes a stronger tincture. Do not pack down. Pour in boiling water to just dampen. (This step is optional, but helps to draw out the beneficial properties of the herbs.) Fill the rest of the jar with glycerine and stir with a clean spoon. **Note:** Glycerine should make up more than half the mixture to adequately preserve the tincture. Cap tightly and let rest in a cool, dark place for 6 to 8 weeks, shaking occasionally.

Pour through a strainer into small jars or tincture vials. Discard the solids. Cap tightly and store in a cool, dark place for up to 1 year.

Optional Heat Step

Make the mixture as instructed above but instead of storing for 6 to 8 weeks, use heat to speed up the process. Place a washcloth or silicone baking mat (to keep jar from breaking) in the bottom of a slow cooker. Fill the cooker up with water to cover three-quarters of the jar (don't cover the lid!) and turn on the "keep warm" or lowest setting. Keep in the slow cooker for at least 1 day on this setting, adding water as needed (I've let it go for 2 days). Let cool, strain, and store as usual.

Chamomile "Rest and Relax" Glycerite

¾ cup chamomile flowers

Boiling water

1 cup + 2 tablespoons food-grade vegetable glycerine, plus more if needed

Place the flowers in a pint-size mason jar. Pour in boiling water to just dampen. (This step is optional but helps to draw out the beneficial properties of the herbs.) Fill the rest of the jar with glycerine and stir with a clean spoon. **Note:** Glycerine should make up more than half of the mixture to adequately preserve the tincture. Cap tightly and let rest in a cool, dark place for 6 to 8 weeks, shaking occasionally. Or, use optional heat step (see page 154), if desired, to speed up the process.

Pour through a strainer into small jars or tincture vials. Discard the solids. Cap tightly and store in a cool, dry place.

Plantain "Tummy Soothe" Glycerite

¾ cup dried plantain leaf

Boiling water

1 cup + 2 tablespoons food-grade vegetable glycerine, plus more if needed

Place the plantain leaf in a pint-size mason jar. Pour in just enough boiling water to dampen. (This step is optional but helps to draw out the beneficial properties of the herbs.) Fill the rest of the jar with glycerine and stir with a clean spoon. **Note:** Glycerine should make up more than half of the mixture to adequately preserve the tincture. Cap tightly and let rest in a cool dark place for 6 to 8 weeks, shaking occasionally. Or, use optional heat step (page 154), if desired, to speed up the process.

Pour through a strainer into small jars or tincture vials. Discard the solids. Cap tightly and store in a cool, dry place.

St. John's Wort "Calm and Happy" Glycerite

¾ cup St. John's wort

Boiling water

1 cup + 2 tablespoons food-grade vegetable glycerine, plus more if needed

Place the St. John's wort in a pint-size mason jar. Pour in just enough boiling water to dampen. (This step is optional but helps to draw out the beneficial properties of the herbs.) Fill the rest of the jar with glycerine and stir with a clean spoon. **Note:** Glycerine should make up more than half of the mixture to adequately preserve the tincture. Cap tightly and let rest in a cool, dark place for 6 to 8 weeks, shaking occasionally. Or, use optional heat step (page 154), if desired, to speed up the process.

Pour through a strainer into small jars or tincture vials. Discard the solids. Cap tightly and store in a cool, dry place.

Valerian "Calm Sleep" Glycerite

¾ cup dried valerian root

Boiling water

1 cup + 2 tablespoons food-grade vegetable glycerine, plus more if needed

Place the valerian in a pint-size mason jar. Pour in just enough boiling water to dampen. (This step is optional but helps to draw out the beneficial properties of the herbs.) Fill the rest of the jar with glycerine and stir with a clean spoon. **Note:** Glycerine should make up more than half of the mixture to adequately preserve the tincture. Cap tightly and let rest in a cool, dark place for 6 to 8 weeks, shaking occasionally. Or, use optional heat step (page 154), if desired, to speed up the process.

Pour through a strainer into small jars or tincture vials. Discard the solids. Cap tightly and store in a cool, dry place.

Mom-to-Be Glycerite

¼ cup dried red raspberry leaf

¼ cup dried nettle leaf

¼ cup dried alfalfa leaf

Boiling water

1 cup + 2 tablespoons food-grade vegetable glycerine, plus more if needed

Place the herbs in a pint-size mason jar. Pour in just enough boiling water to dampen. (This step is optional but helps to draw out the beneficial properties of the herbs.) Fill the rest of the jar (or the entire jar if not using hot water too) with glycerine and stir with a clean spoon. **Note:** Glycerine should make up more than half of the mixture to adequately preserve the tincture. Cap tightly and let rest in a cool, dark place for 6 to 8 weeks, shaking occasionally. Or, use optional heat step (page 154), if desired, to speed up the process.

Pour through a strainer into small jars or tincture vials. Discard the solids. Cap tightly and store in a cool, dry place.

Plantain Poultice for Itchy or Sunburned Skin

3 tablespoons dried plantain leaf
1 tablespoon bentonite clay
Boiling water

In a small glass bowl, mix together the plantain powder and clay. Pour in just enough boiling water to make a thick paste. Let cool slightly.

Cut a 1-square-foot piece of cheesecloth. Spread the paste between two layers of the cloth and fold over the edges.

To use, apply the poultice to the wound. (Wrap in waterproof material first if desired.) Leave on for 15 minutes to 2 hours, or as needed.

Activated Charcoal Poultice for Spider Bites

3 tablespoons activated charcoal powder
Boiling water

Place the activated charcoal in a small glass bowl and pour in just enough boiling water to make a thick paste. Let cool slightly.

Cut a 1-square-foot piece of cheesecloth. Spread the paste between two layers of the cloth and fold over the edges.

To use, apply the poultice to the wound. (Wrap in waterproof material first if desired.) Leave on for 15 minutes to 2 hours, or as needed.

Baking Soda Poultice for Skin Wounds

This poultice is great for minor bug bites and minor itchy skin or irritation.

  3 tablespoons baking soda
  Boiling water

Place the baking soda in a small glass bowl and pour in just enough boiling water to make a thick paste. Let cool slightly.

Cut a 1-square-foot piece of cheesecloth. Spread the paste between two layers of the cloth and fold over the edges.

To use, apply the poultice to the wound. (Wrap in waterproof material first if desired.) Leave on for 15 minutes to 2 hours, or as needed.

Onion Poultice for Skin Wounds

  ¼ yellow onion, thinly sliced
  Boiling water

Place the onion in a small saucepan with 2 tablespoons water and sauté over medium heat until the water evaporates and the onion slightly wilts, 2 to 3 minutes. Remove from the heat and place the onion slices between two layers of cheesecloth and fold over the edges.

To use, apply to the wound. (Wrap in waterproof material first if desired.) Leave on for 15 minutes to 2 hours, or as needed.

Cabbage Poultice

Use this poultice to ease the pain of breast engorgement.

3 garlic cloves
2 cabbage leaves, washed

Thinly slice garlic cloves and place them between the cabbage leaves. The cabbage can be applied directly to the skin, but if you prefer, place them between two layers of cheesecloth and fold over the edges.

To use, apply the poultice to the skin and leave on for 1 to 2 hours, or as needed. For mastitis, I place the cabbage leaves directly in my bra and change them out as needed.

Garlic "Warts Be Gone" Poultice

1 clove garlic

Using a mortar and pestle, mash the garlic with a tiny amount of water to make a paste. Spoon a small amount of the paste directly on the wart, being careful to avoid healthy skin around the wart. Cover tightly with a bandage and leave on for up to 1 hour. Repeat this process daily for 2 weeks to help remove the wart.

Clay Poultice for Splinters

3 tablespoons bentonite clay
Boiling water

Place the clay in a small glass bowl and pour in just enough boiling water to make a thick paste. Let cool slightly.

Cut a 1-square-foot piece of cheesecloth. Spread the paste between two layers of the cloth and fold over the edges.

To use, apply the poultice to the area with the splinter. (Wrap in waterproof material first if desired.) Leave on for 15 minutes to 2 hours, or as needed.

Salt Poultice for Skin Wounds

3 tablespoons sea salt
Boiling water

Place the salt in a small glass bowl and pour in just enough boiling water to make a thick paste. Let cool slightly.

Cut a 1-square-foot piece of cheesecloth. Spread the paste between two layers of the cloth and fold over the edges.

To use, apply the poultice to the wound. (Wrap in waterproof material first if desired.) Leave on for 15 minutes to 2 hours, or as needed.

Magnesium Poultice for Relaxation and Sore Muscles

3 tablespoons magnesium chloride flakes
Boiling water

Place the magnesium flakes in a small glass bowl and pour in just enough boiling water to make a thick paste. Let cool slightly.

Cut a 1-square-foot piece of cheesecloth. Spread the paste between two layers of the cloth and fold over the edges.

To use, apply the poultice to sore muscles or to the bottom of feet for relaxation. (Wrap in waterproof material first if desired.) Leave on for 15 minutes to 2 hours, or as needed.

Plantain and Dandelion Eczema Poultice

3 tablespoons dried plantain leaf
2 tablespoons dried dandelion leaf
Boiling water

In a blender or mini–food processor, blend the herbs until powdered. Pour in just enough boiling water to make a thick paste and blend again. Let cool slightly.

Cut a 1-square-foot piece of cheesecloth. Spread the paste between two layers of the cloth and fold over the edges.

To use, apply to the affected area of skin. (Wrap in waterproof material first if desired.) Leave on for 15 minutes to 2 hours, or as needed.

Elderberry Hemorrhoid Poultice

3 tablespoons dried elderberries
Boiling water

In a blender or mini–food processor, blend the elderberries with just enough boiling water to make a thick paste. Let cool slightly.

Cut a 1-square-foot piece of cheesecloth. Spread the paste between two layers of the cloth and fold over the edges.

To use, apply to the affected area. Leave on for 15 minutes to 2 hours, or as needed.

Slippery Elm Sore Joint Poultice

3 tablespoons dried slippery elm
Boiling water

Place the slippery elm in a small glass bowl and pour in just enough boiling water to make a thick paste. Let cool slightly.

Cut a 1-square-foot piece of cheesecloth. Spread the paste between two layers of the cloth and fold over the edges.

To use, apply to sore joints. Leave on for 15 minutes to 2 hours, or as needed.

Skin Care Recipes

Tamanu Castor Oil Cleansing Blend for Oily Skin

Castor oil is considered more drying than other oils, so this blend tends to work best on oily skin.

2 tablespoons castor oil

¼ cup sunflower oil

1 teaspoon tamanu oil (optional)

10 drops patchouli essential oil (optional)

Pour the castor oil, sunflower oil, and (if using) the tamanu oil and patchouli essential oil into a small glass dropper bottle. To use, see "Steps for Oil Cleansing" on page 57.

Argan Lavender Oil Cleansing Blend for Combination Skin

Argan and lavender help balance the skin's natural oils in this combination blend.

1 tablespoon castor oil

¼ cup sunflower oil or olive oil

1 teaspoon argan oil (optional)

10 drops lavender essential oil (optional)

Pour the castor oil, sunflower oil, and (if using) the argan oil and lavender essential oil into a small glass dropper bottle. To use, see "Steps for Oil Cleansing" on page 57.

Not a fan of putting oil on your face? No problem. There are some great simple recipes for foaming cleansers as well. Just pick the best option for your skin type and feel free to customize to get your perfect blend.

Olive and Neroli Oil Cleansing Blend for Dry Skin

Olive oil and neroli essential oil deeply nourish the skin while cleansing gently to avoid drying.

 ¼ cup olive oil
 1 teaspoon castor oil
 10 drops neroli essential oil (optional)

Pour the olive oil, castor oil, and (if using) the neroli essential oil into a small glass dropper bottle. To use, see "Steps for Oil Cleansing" on page 57.

Foaming Witch Hazel Facial Cleanser for Oily Skin

Witch hazel is naturally astringent and great for minimizing pores and reducing overproduction of oil. When combined with the other ingredients in this cleanser, it helps to nourish and cleanse skin without adding excess oil.

$^2/_3$ cup liquid castile soap, such as Dr. Bronner's

30 drops melaleuca essential oil

30 drops lavender essential oil

10 drops sea buckthorn oil or rosehip oil

About $^1/_3$ cup witch hazel

Pour the castile soap, both essential oils, and the sea buckthorn oil into an 8-ounce or larger liquid soap pump dispenser. Swirl the bottle until they are well combined. Add the witch hazel, leaving at least 1 inch of space at the top for the pump. You may not need the full ⅓ cup to fill the dispenser. If the castile soap is thin, then reduce the witch hazel to ¼ cup.

Cap the dispenser tightly and gently tip it back and forth to mix everything. Don't shake it too much, though, or you'll have a bunch of suds!

Foaming Chamomile Avocado Facial Cleanser for Dry Skin

This blend has nourishing avocado oil to step up the moisturizing. Avocado oil provides moisture while essential oils help restore balance.

$\frac{2}{3}$ cup liquid castile soap, such as Dr. Bronner's

30 drops frankincense essential oil

30 drops lavender essential oil

1 teaspoon avocado oil

About $\frac{1}{3}$ cup chamomile hydrosol

Pour the castile soap, both essential oils, and the avocado oil into a liquid soap pump dispenser. Swirl the bottle until they are well combined. Add the hydrosol, leaving at least 1 inch of space at the top for the pump. You may not need the full ⅓ cup to fill it. If the castile soap is thin, then reduce the hydrosol to ¼ cup.

Cap the dispenser tightly and gently tip it back and forth to mix everything. Don't shake it too much, though, or you'll have a bunch of suds!

Foaming Patchouli Almond Facial Cleanser for Normal Skin

Have normal skin? Lucky you! This cleanser works on almost all skin types but is best for normal or combination skin.

2/3 cup liquid castile soap, such as Dr. Bronner's

30 drops patchouli essential oil

10 drops orange essential oil

2 teaspoons almond oil

About 1/3 cup cucumber hydrosol

Pour the castile soap, both essential oils, and the almond oil into a liquid soap pump dispenser. Swirl the bottle until they are well combined. Add the hydrosol, leaving at least 1 inch of space at the top for the pump. You may not need the full 1/3 cup to fill it. If the castile soap is thin, then reduce the hydrosol to 1/4 cup.

Cap the dispenser tightly and gently tip it back and forth to mix everything. Don't shake it too much, though, or you'll have a bunch of suds!

Lavender and Honey Face Wash

Did you know that honey makes a wonderful face wash? It nourishes skin, tightens pores, and kills bacteria. For this, make sure to use a high-quality raw honey, preferably a manuka honey.

¼ cup raw honey, preferably manuka

20 drops lavender essential oil

Mix together the honey and lavender in a small glass jar. To use, wet down your face and neck with warm water and massage 1 teaspoon face wash into your skin in a circular motion. Leave on for 5 minutes and rinse well with a warm, wet washcloth.

Oatmeal-Lavender Soothing Facial Scrub

Need some exfoliation? This gentle oatmeal facial scrub exfoliates skin naturally with lavender and oatmeal plus salt and baking soda for gentle scrubbing.

½ cup rolled oats
10 drops lavender essential oil
1 tablespoon lavender flowers
1 tablespoon baking soda
1 tablespoon fine sea salt

Place the oats, essential oil, and flowers in a coffee grinder and pulse until ground, 45 to 60 seconds. (A blender can also be used, but a coffee grinder is the preferred option here.) Transfer to a small bowl and stir in the baking soda and salt. Store the face scrub in a tightly capped small glass jar.

To use, combine 2 teaspoons scrub with 1½ teaspoons water or milk, then gently scrub across the face with the fingers.

Tips for Using the Facial Scrub

- The scrub can also be mixed with aloe vera or honey, both of which soothe, rejuvenate, and calm the skin.
- The scrub also works well as a mask. Simply mix the scrub with the desired liquid until it's a thick paste, and smooth over the skin. Leave on for 10 to 20 minutes, then rinse off with warm water.

Basic Sugar Scrub

Sugar isn't great for the body when ingested, but it is wonderful for the skin, especially when combined with nourishing oils to make an exfoliating scrub. You can make endless variations of sugar scrubs by mixing 4 parts sugar to 1 part oil and adding any scents you like.

1 cup organic cane sugar
¼ cup almond oil
10 drops essential oil of choice (optional)

In a small glass bowl, mix together the sugar, almond oil, and (if using) the essential oil until combined. Store in a small, tightly capped glass jar in a cool, dark place for up to 6 months.

To use, scoop out a small amount of sugar scrub and gently rub into the skin in a circular motion to exfoliate. Rinse well.

Chai Latte Sugar Scrub

Enjoy the antioxidant benefits of cinnamon in this soothing chai-scented scrub.

1 cup organic cane sugar
¼ cup unrefined coconut oil
1 tablespoon ground cinnamon
½ teaspoon ground ginger
2 drops clove essential oil

In a small glass bowl, mix together all the ingredients until combined. Store in a small, tightly capped glass jar in a cool, dark place for up to 6 months.

To use, scoop out a small amount of sugar scrub and gently rub into the skin in a circular motion to exfoliate. Rinse well.

Lavender-Lemon Olive Oil–Sugar Scrub

A relaxing and clarifying scrub with notes of lavender and lemon.

    1 cup organic cane sugar
    ¼ cup olive oil
    10 drops lavender essential oil
    5 drops lemon essential oil

In a small glass bowl, mix together all the ingredients until combined. Store in a small, tightly capped glass jar in a cool, dark place for up to 6 months.

To use, scoop out a small amount of sugar scrub and gently rub into the skin in a circular motion. Rinse well.

Himalayan Mint and Grapefruit Salt Scrub

An exfoliating scrub with grapefruit and mint in a salt base. Great for making skin silky and firm.

    1 cup finely ground Himalayan salt
    3 tablespoons olive oil
    1 tablespoon liquid castile soap, such as Dr. Bronner's
    30 drops grapefruit essential oil
    2 drops peppermint essential oil

In a small glass bowl, mix together all the ingredients until combined. Store in a small, tightly capped glass jar in a cool, dark place for up to 6 months.

To use, scoop out a small amount of salt scrub and gently rub into the skin in a circular motion. Rinse well.

Cooling Magnesium Mint Sea Spray Toner

A mineral-rich spray toner helps balance all skin types.

   1 cup boiling distilled water

   1 tablespoon sea salt

   Epsom salts (optional)

   1 teaspoon magnesium flakes

   5 drops peppermint essential oil (optional)

Pour the boiling water into a small glass bowl, add the salt, the Epsom salts (if using), and the magnesium flakes and stir until completely dissolved. Stir in the essential oil (if using). Store in a small, tightly capped glass jar or spray bottle in a cool, dark place for up to 6 months.

To use, spray or pour a small amount on a cotton pad and apply to the skin as a toner. It is effective for use as part of a daily skin care routine.

Vitamin C Serum

   $\frac{1}{2}$ teaspoon natural real-food vitamin C powder

   1 tablespoon distilled water or 1 teaspoon distilled water + 2 tablespoons vegetable glycerine (see Note)

In a glass measuring cup, dissolve the vitamin C powder in the water. Store in a tightly capped, dark-colored glass container (vitamin C oxidizes easily) in the refrigerator for up to 1 week. (If using glycerine, dissolve the vitamin C powder in the water-glycerine mixture and store. This version will last up to 2 weeks in the refrigerator.)

Note: Personally, I prefer the vitamin C and water recipe as a toner after cleansing, although glycerine is moisturizing and softening for the skin and will keep longer. Never use glycerine for oral care because it is bad for teeth.

Foaming Lime Body Wash

This body wash is great for all skin types and is super simple to make!

  3 tablespoons liquid castile soap

  3 tablespoons raw honey

  1 tablespoon castor oil

  1 tablespoon olive oil

  10 drops lime essential oil

In a small glass bowl, mix together all the ingredients until combined. Transfer to a liquid soap pump dispenser and use as a body wash.

Unscented Luxurious Oil-Based Lotion

This oil-based recipe is very moisturizing and thick. If you're looking for a lighter, smoother recipe, use Basic Emulsified Lotion (page 179).

½ cup almond or olive oil
¼ cup unrefined coconut oil
¼ cup beeswax
2 tablespoons shea butter

In a pint-size mason jar, mix together all the ingredients and loosely cap. (Alternately, you can use a glass bowl over a saucepan as a double boiler.) I have a mason jar that I keep just for making lotions and lotion bars, or you can even reuse a glass jar from pickles, olives, or other foods.

Fill a medium saucepan with 2 inches water and place over medium heat. Place the jar in the saucepan. As the water heats, the lotion mixture will start to melt. Gently shake or stir occasionally to incorporate.

When the lotion is completely melted, carefully pour it into 8-ounce mason jars or other small tins for storage. It will not pump well in a lotion pump!

Use as you would regular lotion. This has a longer shelf life than some homemade lotion recipes since all the ingredients are already shelf stable and no water is added. Use within 6 months for the best moisturizing benefits.

TIP: A little goes a long way! This lotion is incredibly nourishing and is also great for diaper rash on baby, eczema, and preventing stretch marks!

Chamomile-Calendula Lotion for Kids

½ cup almond or olive oil infused with chamomile and calendula (see page 50)

¼ cup unrefined coconut oil

¼ cup beeswax

1 teaspoon vitamin E oil

2 tablespoons shea butter or cocoa butter

10 drops lavender essential oil (optional)

In a pint-size mason jar, mix together the almond oil, coconut oil, beeswax, vitamin E oil, shea butter, and (if using) the lavender essential oil and loosely cap. (Alternately, you can use a glass bowl over a saucepan as a double boiler.)

Fill a medium saucepan with 2 inches water and place over medium heat. Place the jar in the saucepan. As the water heats, the lotion mixture will start to melt. Shake or stir occasionally to incorporate.

When completely melted, carefully pour into 8-ounce mason jars or other small tins for storage. It will not pump well in a lotion pump!

Use as you would regular lotion. This has a longer shelf life than some homemade lotion recipes since all the ingredients are already shelf stable and no water is added. Use within 6 months for best moisturizing benefits.

Tip: I have a mason jar that I keep just for making lotions and lotion bars, or you can even reuse a glass jar from pickles, olives, or other foods.

Mint and Green Tea Antioxidant Lotion

½ cup almond or olive oil infused with peppermint leaf (see page 50)

¼ cup beeswax

½ teaspoon dried matcha green tea powder

1 teaspoon vitamin E oil (optional)

2 tablespoons shea or cocoa butter (optional)

10 drops essential oil of choice or 1 teaspoon vanilla or other natural extract (optional)

In a pint-size mason jar, mix together the almond oil, beeswax, matcha, and (if using) the vitamin E oil, shea butter, and essential oil and loosely cap. (Alternately, you can use a glass bowl over a saucepan as a double boiler.)

Fill a medium saucepan with 2 inches water and place over medium heat. Place the jar in the saucepan. As the water heats, the lotion mixture will start to melt. Shake or stir occasionally to incorporate.

When completely melted, carefully pour into 8-ounce mason jars or other small tins for storage. It will not pump well in a lotion pump! Use within 6 months.

Basic Emulsified Lotion

⅔ cup almond or grapeseed oil

2 tablespoons unrefined coconut oil

2 tablespoons shea butter

1 tablespoon emulsifying wax

⅔ cup hydrosol, aloe vera gel, or water

In a double boiler over low heat, melt the almond oil, coconut oil, shea butter, and emulsifying wax. Remove to a food processor and let cool slightly. Add the hydrosol one drop at a time while blending until completely incorporated. Use within 1 month.

Rosewater Almond Oil Lotion

⅔ cup almond oil

2 tablespoons coconut oil

2 tablespoons shea butter

1 tablespoon beeswax

⅔ cup rosewater

10 drops lavender essential oil (optional)

In a double boiler over low heat, melt the almond oil, coconut oil, shea butter, and beeswax in a double boiler. Remove to a food processor and let cool slightly. Add the rosewater one drop at a time and lavender essential oil, if using, while blending until completely incorporated. Use within one month.

Grapefruit and Ginger Cellulite Lotion

⅔ cup dried ginger infused oil (see page 50)

2 tablespoons unrefined coconut oil

2 tablespoons shea butter

1 tablespoon beeswax

⅔ cup hydrosol, aloe vera gel, or water

10 drops grapefruit essential oil

In a double boiler over low heat, melt the ginger oil, coconut oil, shea butter, and beeswax. Remove to a food processor and let cool slightly. Add the hydrosol one drop at a time with the grapefruit essential oil, if using, while blending until completely incorporated. Use within 1 month.

Lavender and Vanilla Lotion

⅔ cup almond or grapeseed oil

2 tablespoons unrefined coconut oil

2 tablespoons shea butter

1 tablespoon beeswax

⅔ cup hydrosol, aloe vera gel, or water

1 tablespoon pure vanilla extract

15 drops lavender essential oil

In a double boiler over low heat, melt the almond oil, coconut oil, shea butter, and beeswax. Remove to a food processor and let cool slightly. Add the hydrosol and vanilla extract one drop at a time with the lavender oil, if using, while blending until completely incorporated. Use within 1 month.

Basic Lotion Bars

Easy-to-make lotion bars are incredibly nourishing on dry skin. This recipe can be adjusted to make any quantity that you'd like. I made with equal 1 cup measurements. The recipe I used made exactly 12 lotion bars with my molds. For a small batch, this recipe could be cut in half or even one fourth.

1 cup unrefined coconut oil
1 cup shea butter, cocoa butter, or mango butter or equal parts of each
1 cup beeswax
1 teaspoon vitamin E oil (optional)
20+ drops essential oil of choice (optional)

In a double boiler over low heat, melt the coconut oil, shea butter, beeswax, and (if using) vitamin E oil (see Tip). Remove from the heat and add the essential oil (if using). Gently stir by hand until the essential oil is incorporated.

Carefully pour into lotion bar tubes or silicone molds (see Tip). A square baking pan also works. Allow the lotion bars to cool completely before attempting to pop out of molds. If you've used a baking pan, simply cut into whatever size bars you'd like.

TIP: I found an old double boiler at a thrift store that I use for skin products only.
These lotion bars can be made in different molds for holiday gifts—hearts for Valentine's Day, flowers for Mother's Day, egg or bunny molds for Easter.

Geranium Shea Moisturizing Lotion Bars

2 tablespoons raw organic shea butter

1 tablespoon unrefined coconut oil, solid at room temp
(can use extra shea butter if allergic to coconut)

2 teaspoons olive oil or castor oil

2 teaspoons beeswax

20 drops geranium essential oil

In a double boiler over low heat, melt the shea butter, coconut oil, olive oil, and beeswax. Remove from the heat and add the essential oil. Pour into lotion bar tubes or silicone molds. Let cool for several hours or overnight. I put mine in the refrigerator to speed the cooling process.

Basic Body Butter

$\frac{1}{2}$ cup shea butter

$\frac{1}{2}$ cup cocoa butter or mango butter

$\frac{1}{2}$ cup unrefined coconut oil

$\frac{1}{2}$ cup light oil, such as almond, jojoba, or olive

10 to 30 drops essential oil of choice (optional)

In a double boiler over medium heat, melt both butters, the coconut oil, and the light oil, stirring constantly. Remove from the heat, stir in essential oils, and let cool slightly, then place in the refrigerator and chill until starting to harden but still somewhat soft, about 1 hour.

Remove from the refrigerator. Using a hand mixer, whip until fluffy, about 10 minutes. Return to the refrigerator for 10 to 15 minutes to set.

Transfer the lotion to a pint-size mason jar, cap tightly, and store. Use as you would regular lotion or body butter.

NOTE: If your home stays above 75°F, the lotion may become too soft and need to be kept in the refrigerator.

Magnesium-Infused Body Butter

½ cup magnesium flakes + 3 tablespoons boiling water,
   or ½ cup premade magnesium-infused oil
¼ cup unrefined coconut oil
2 tablespoons emulsifying wax or beeswax (but beeswax is more difficult to mix)
3 tablespoons shea butter

In a small glass bowl, mix together the magnesium flakes and boiling water until dissolved. This will create a thick liquid. Set aside to cool.

In a quart-size mason jar, combine the coconut oil, emulsifying wax, and shea butter and loosely cap.

Fill a medium saucepan with 2 inches water and place over medium heat. Place the jar in the saucepan. As the water heats, the lotion mixture will start to melt. Shake or stir occasionally to incorporate.

When completely melted, remove the jar from the pan and let the mixture cool to room temperature. It should be slightly opaque.

Pour the mixture into a medium glass bowl. Using a hand mixer or immersion blender on medium speed, blend the oil mixture. Slowly (starting with a drop at a time), while blending, add the dissolved magnesium to the oil mixture until all the magnesium mix is added and it is well incorporated. Place in the refrigerator for 15 minutes, then remove and reblend to a buttery consistency.

Store in a clean quart-size mason jar in the refrigerator for a cooling lotion (best consistency) or at room temp for up to 2 months.

Hand soap often costs several dollars at the store, but you can make a natural version in just minutes and for under a tenth of the price! Reuse whatever container you have to reduce waste. If you already use a foaming hand soap, use the foaming soap recipe below to replace it. If you prefer a liquid soap, use the liquid recipe.

Sea-Fresh Foaming Hand Soap

2 tablespoons liquid castile soap (I like using scented ones)

½ teaspoon olive or almond oil (optional)

5 drops lavender essential oil

4 drops bergamot essential oil

2 drops rosemary essential oil

1 drop eucalyptus essential oil

Fill a large liquid soap pump dispenser with 2 ounces water. You'll want to leave about 1 inch of space at the top for the pump. Add the castile soap to the water mixture (do not add the soap first or it will create bubbles when the water is added). Add the olive oil (if using; it does help preserve the life of the dispenser) and the essential oils.

Cap the dispenser tightly and lightly swish to mix. Use as you would any regular foaming soap.

Fresh and Clean Liquid Hand Soap

1 ounce finely grated bar unscented soap

5 drops lavender essential oil

5 drops lemon essential oil

2 drops rosemary essential oil

Place the bar soap and 1 quart water in a medium saucepan over medium heat. Stir constantly until the soap has dissolved. Remove from the heat and let cool completely. Add the essential oils, mixing well to incorporate. Store in a quart-size mason jar for up to 1 month.

Note: It will take about 24 hours for the soap to completely gel; it will not be quite as thick as regular hand soap. You can add more grated bar soap to create a thicker soap, but it will be more difficult to pump and will not get hands any more clean, so I stick with this. After 24 hours, shake well to make sure it has gelled completely and use as usual.

Bentonite Mask for the Skin

I apply a paste of bentonite clay and water on skin irritations like blemishes, insect bites, cuts, skin itching, or burns. I leave it on until it dries and then I wash it off. This is said to be especially calming for eczema, psoriasis, chicken pox, and so forth.

Bentonite Poultice for Bites, Burns, Cuts, and Stings

For more severe issues, I create a poultice by putting a thick layer of bentonite clay on the skin and applying a wet gauze or cloth over it. I wrap the area and leave the poultice on, changing every 2 hours.

Bentonite Face Mask

For smooth and healthy skin, I make a paste of bentonite clay and water and apply to my face as a mask. (A similar mask is used in many spas.) I leave it on for 20 minutes and wash off. I typically do this once or twice a week.

Deep-Cleansing Mud Mask

Bentonite clay, honey, and herbs come together for a mask that works deep into pores to cleanse and tighten.

1 teaspoon bentonite clay
½ teaspoon each ground chamomile and lavender (optional)
1 teaspoon raw honey
10 drops lavender essential oil (optional)

In a small glass bowl, mix together the clay and (if using) herbs. Add the honey and stir until a thick paste forms. Thin the paste by stirring in 1 teaspoon water, or more if needed. Stir in the essential oil (if using).

To use, immediately apply to the face and neck in a circular motion, avoiding the eyes. Leave on for 10 to 15 minutes, or until it has hardened. Wash off with a dark-colored washcloth soaked in hot water (really hot water helps to steam off the mask without having to rub the skin). Pat your face dry and enjoy your smooth skin!

Probiotic Cooling Yogurt Mask

Did you know that the skin has a microbiome just like the gut does? Harsh cleansers and other chemical exposure can strip important bacteria from the skin. Help give your skin its probiotics back with this cooling mask.

1 tablespoon whole milk organic plain yogurt

1 capsule probiotic powder

1 teaspoon raw honey

Mix together all the ingredients in a small glass bowl and apply to the face. Leave on for 10 to 20 minutes, then rinse with warm water.

Green Tea Antioxidant Mask

This mask is antioxidant rich and leaves skin feeling smooth and firm. My kids call it my ogre mask because my face turns green when I'm wearing it.

1 teaspoon matcha green tea powder

1 teaspoon raw honey

1 teaspoon bentonite clay

In a small glass bowl, mix together all the ingredients with 1 teaspoon water to form a paste. Brush onto the face in a circular motion. Leave on for 5 minutes, then rinse in warm water.

Fizzy Fresh Bath Bomb

Bath bombs are a great way to relax in the tub after a long day of dealing with kids, cooking, and all the other activities that parenthood entails. If you've never tried them, I highly encourage it, as it's one of my favorite things to do at the end of the day.

1 cup baking soda

½ cup citric acid

½ cup sea salt or Epsom salts

¾ cup cornstarch

2 tablespoons carrier oil of choice (olive oil is my personal favorite but any liquid oil will work)

2 teaspoons witch hazel or water, plus a little more in a spray bottle if needed

1 teaspoon pure vanilla extract or water

30 to 40 drops essential oil or ground herbs (ginger is great) (optional)

In a large glass bowl, mix together the baking soda, citric acid, salt, and cornstarch until well combined.

In a small glass bowl, stir together the carrier oil, witch hazel, and vanilla extract. Stir in the essential oil (if using). If you're using ground herbs, do not add yet.

Add the liquid ingredients to the dry a little at a time. Mix well with hands (wear gloves if you have sensitive skin). Add the ground herbs (if using) and mix in well.

The mixture should hold together when squeezed without crumbling. You may need to spray with a little more witch hazel if it hasn't achieved this consistency yet. (Using a spray bottle helps to add the liquid evenly).

Quickly and firmly press the mixture into molds, greased muffin tins, or any other greased container. (Using metal molds will create a stronger and more effective bath bomb.) Let rest for at least 24 hours (48 is better), or until hardened. It will expand some and this is normal. You can push it down into the mold several times while it is drying to keep the mixture from expanding too much. When hardened and dry, remove from the molds and store in an airtight container. Use within 2 weeks.

Powdered Mineral Foundation

At the recommendation of a friend who had used cocoa powder as a natural bronzer, I started experimenting with natural foundation options and came up with a recipe similar to a mineral makeup.

I start with a base of arrowroot powder and zinc oxide (you can also use cornstarch, but arrowroot works better) and then slowly add in cocoa powder and finely ground cinnamon powder until you get a shade close to your skin tone. You can then store in a jar or old powder container and use a brush to apply. It took me a few tries of mixing to get the color correct for my skin tone, but most days a quick brush of this is all I need. I later discovered that adding gold mica powder gave it an even smoother texture and made my skin radiant. Here is the recipe.

> 2 tablespoons zinc oxide or arrowroot powder (the zinc oxide offers better coverage)
> 1 tablespoon arrowroot powder (optional)
> 1/2 to 1 teaspoon white cosmetic, fuller's earth, or French green clay (optional)
> 1 teaspoon gold mica powder
> Up to 1 teaspoon finely ground cocoa powder, bronze mica powder, or a combination
>   of the two to get desired color
> 1 teaspoon translucent mica dust (especially recommended for very oily skin) (optional)

In a small glass bowl, mix together the 2 tablespoons zinc oxide, 1 tablespoon arrowroot (if using), clay, cocoa powder, and mica powder (if using) to get desired color and coverage.

The zinc oxide provides coverage and matte finish. Colored mica powders, natural clays, and cocoa powder will give color. Start slowly and add as needed, testing on the inner arm to find desired shade. Store in a tightly capped small glass jar for up to 1 month.

Note: If you prefer, just arrowroot powder (or white cosmetic clay), cocoa powder, and (optional) cinnamon powder can be used. This will create a great and completely natural/edible foundation, but it will not last as long as a powder containing zinc oxide and mica. I personally feel safe using zinc oxide on my skin (non-nano and uncoated) but if you don't, just stick to the arrowroot version.

Homemade Base Moisturizer

There are actually two options for the base of this recipe: the simple way or the DIY way.

For a simpler version, use a natural store-bought moisturizer for the base and add colors and pigments as needed. If you prefer the store-bought option, I recommend using one of these two natural lotions, which both are rated as safe by the Environmental Working Group (and they make your skin feel incredible!): SheaMoisture Raw Shea Chamomile & Argan Oil Baby Lotion or SheaMoisture Olive & Marula Baby Lotion.

The DIY way takes a little more time and requires five ingredients but allows more customization because you're making the base lotion yourself.

Argan oil   Shea butter
Vegetable-based emulsifying wax   Aloe vera gel
Witch hazel

Add to the base for color and coverage:

Zinc oxide powder (non-nano and uncoated) or white cosmetic, kaolin, fuller's earth, or
    bentonite clay
Mica powders in color of choice (I used bronze and gold)
Organic cocoa powder
OR natural store-bought mineral makeup in your color (in place of the 4 preceding ingredients)

Customize to Your Skin Tone

If you're using a natural store-bought mineral makeup base in your skin tone, just add to the store-bought base or Homemade Base Moisturizer until you get the desired color and coverage.

For the homemade version, I recommend making the base lotion (details below) and testing on your skin to make sure you like the coverage and texture. Once you create your custom base, start adding the color powders (clays, mica, cocoa, zinc, etc.) little by little to get the color and coverage you want.

Some tips:

- If you're using zinc oxide (which is used in many mineral makeups and my natural sunscreen), you'll want to add it first for the coverage aspect. I added about five times as much non-nano zinc oxide as other color.
- Add clays and sprinkle them on very lightly to prevent clumping. I found that a tiny bit of French green clay and fuller's earth clay used together helped even out my skin tone.

- Add color slowly (you can't undo this part!). Start by sprinkling tiny amounts of cocoa powder, bronze mica powder, and gold mica powder and mixing until you get a color that works for your skin.
- Test on the inside of your arm for color and consistency before putting it on your face.
- Optional: Add a couple drops of a skin-safe essential oil, like lavender, frankincense, or rose, for scent and added benefit.
- The zinc and clays offer coverage and smoothing; the mica and cocoa add color and bronzing. Add both slowly until the desired color and coverage are reached. Let cool and retest on the inner arm or neck to confirm it is the right color.
- If you want a thicker crème foundation, add slightly more emulsifying wax or shea butter.
- If you prefer smoother/thinner coverage, add slightly less emulsifying wax or shea butter, or increase the aloe vera gel and witch hazel.

Natural Liquid Foundation

After dozens of tries, I finally created a recipe for a liquid foundation that offers coverage and looks amazing on the skin, without looking clownish.

This recipe combines many of my favorite natural skin products, like shea butter and argan oil, along with natural minerals and clays. Once I discovered how to make a good base for this recipe, it was easy to create natural crème blush and concealer as well.

2 teaspoons argan or jojoba oil

1 teaspoon shea butter

½ teaspoon emulsifying wax

1 tablespoon aloe vera gel

1 teaspoon witch hazel

OR 3 tablespoons of natural store-bought lotion (in place of the 5 preceding ingredients)

1 to 4 teaspoons non-nano zinc oxide

½ teaspoon clay of choice (optional)

½ to 1 teaspoon mica powders of choice

¼ to ½ teaspoon cocoa powder

OR 2 to 3 teaspoons of a store-bought natural mineral powder in color of choice (in place of the 4 preceding ingredients)

If making the simple version, just mix the purchased lotion and mineral powder to get the desired color and consistency.

Instructions for the Complete DIY

In a double boiler over medium heat, melt the argan oil, shea butter, and emulsifying wax. Add the aloe vera gel and witch hazel and whisk until completely incorporated and smooth. Remove from the heat.

Slowly, start adding colors. Start with zinc oxide and (if using) the clay until desired coverage is reached. It will still be quite pale at this point. Add the mica and cocoa powders a tiny pinch at a time until desired color is reached.

Dip the tip of a spoon into the mixture. Let cool for a few seconds, then test the color and coverage on your forehead to make sure you've achieved the right tone for your skin.

Spoon the mixture into the desired container and let completely cool. This makeup can be easily stored in a glass jar or old makeup container. My favorite way to store is in a silicone squeezable tube for easy application. This helps prevent contamination since you aren't reaching into the makeup container and it keeps it fresh longer. I prefer to squeeze a small amount onto a makeup sponge and apply. A little goes a long way.

Natural Powder Blush

If you enjoy making your own natural makeup, you're going to want some blush too. Since it's homemade, it's actually good for your skin and won't expose your body to a bevy of toxins.

½ teaspoon arrowroot powder
½ teaspoon cocoa powder
½ teaspoon ground hibiscus

As with any homemade makeup recipe, the amounts vary by person. You'll have to experiment with quantities of each ingredient to find the shade that works for you. I always start with a base of about ½ teaspoon of arrowroot and darken as needed, testing on my inner arm as I go.

When you get your desired shade, store in a small jar or old makeup shaker and use as needed. If you're not a fan of powdered makeup, you can also make a crème version of this same concept.

Crème Blush

The benefit of a crème blush is that it stays on longer and can be much bolder and more versatile than powdered blush. A little goes a really long way. I also use a small amount to darken my natural foundation if I need to during summer months.

I typically use a makeup brush to apply this foundation, but you can also easily use your fingers. The basic ingredients are the same as those for the liquid foundation recipe and there are two options for this recipe: the simple way or the DIY way.

For a simpler version, use a natural store-bought moisturizer for the base and add colors and pigments as needed. If you prefer the store-bought option, these two lotions are both rated as safe by the Environmental Working Group and they make a great base: SheaMoisture Raw Shea Chamomile & Argan Oil Baby Lotion or SheaMoisture Olive & Marula Baby Lotion.

The DIY way takes a little more time and requires three ingredients but allows more customization since you're making the base lotion yourself. For the DIY version, you'll need these ingredients for the base:

- Shea butter
- Vegetable-based emulsifying wax
- Aloe vera gel

Add to the base for color:

- Mica powders in color of choice (I used bronze and pearl red)
- Organic cocoa powder
- OR natural store-bought mineral makeup in your color (in place of the 2 preceding ingredients)

1 teaspoon shea butter

1/2 teaspoon emulsifying wax

1 tablespoon aloe gel

OR 1 tablespoon natural store-bought lotion (in place of the 3 preceding ingredients)

1/2 to 1 teaspoon mica powders of choice

1/2 to 1 teaspoon cocoa powder

OR 1 to 2 teaspoons store-bought natural mineral powder (in place of the 2 preceding ingredients)

If making the simple version, just mix the purchased lotion and mineral powder to get the desired color and consistency.

Instructions for the Complete DIY

In a double boiler over medium heat, melt the shea butter and emulsifying wax. Add the aloe vera gel and whisk until completely incorporated and smooth. Remove from the heat.

Slowly, start adding colors. Add the mica and cocoa powders a tiny pinch at a time until desired color is reached.

Dip the tip of a spoon into the mixture. Let cool for a few seconds, then test the color and coverage on your cheek to make sure you've achieved the right tone for your skin.

Spoon the mixture into the desired container and let cool.

Additional Tips

- Adding colors (mica powders and cocoa powder) to a store-bought lotion will create a very smooth blush/bronzer. Experiment with the colors until you get the desired shade. It will look much darker while making it than it will on skin.
- Making a homemade lotion as a base will give the most options for customizing but is also the most difficult. With the homemade one, adding more vegetable wax will make a thicker and longer lasting blush/bronzer; using more aloe will make a smoother and more subtle mix.
- Adding more reddish mica powders will give a more rosy-pink hue like a blush; more cocoa powder or bronze mica will create a bronzer or more tan mixture.

Herbal Hair Detox for Blonde Hair

¼ cup chamomile flowers

2 tablespoons nettle leaf

2 cups boiling water

½ cup plus 1 tablespoon apple cider vinegar

About ¾ cup bentonite or redmond clay

5 drops rosemary essential oil

Brew a strong tea to use as the base liquid for this recipe: Place the flowers and nettle in a small nonmetal bowl, pour in the boiling water, and let steep until cool, about 10 minutes. Chamomile helps brighten light-colored hair and nettle is great for hair growth.

Pour through a strainer into a glass jar. Discard the solids. Reserve 1 cup tea in the jar. Add 1 tablespoon vinegar and set aside to use as a final rinse in the shower (if desired).

Pour the tea and ½ cup vinegar into a blender. (Alternatively, you can whisk together the ingredients in a nonmetal bowl.) Add the clay 1 tablespoon at a time while blending to incorporate it. Keep adding clay until the mixture is smooth and about the consistency of yogurt. Blend in the essential oil.

Store in a tightly capped container in the shower for up to 1 week.

To Use: Wet your hair. Starting at the roots, massage a handful of the clay mixture into hair and work down to the roots. Repeat until all hair is coated. Leave for 5 to 20 minutes—but do not let dry! Rinse out with warm water.

Optional: Rinse with the 1 cup reserved herb-vinegar tea.

Note: Bentonite clay is most effective if it doesn't come in contact with metal prior to use. Mix the ingredients in a wood, plastic, or glass bowl for best results, though I haven't found that this makes much of a difference for hair products. Don't want to use your kitchen blender for hair products? I use an old mini–food processor with a plastic dough blade that I found at a thrift shop.

Herbal Hair Detox for Brown or Black Hair

¼ cup dried rosemary

2 tablespoons dried nettle leaf

2 cups boiling water

½ cup apple cider vinegar

About ¾ cup bentonite or redmond clay

5 drops rosemary essential oil

Brew a strong tea to use as the base liquid for this recipe: Place the rosemary and nettle in a small nonmetal bowl, pour in the boiling water, and let steep until cool, about 10 minutes. Rosemary helps brighten light-colored hair and nettle is great for hair growth.

Pour through a strainer into a glass jar. Discard the solids. Reserve 1 cup in the jar. Add 1 tablespoon vinegar and set aside to use as a final rinse in the shower (if desired).

Pour the tea and ½ cup vinegar into a blender. (Alternatively, you can whisk together the ingredients in a nonmetal bowl.) Add the clay 1 tablespoon at a time while blending to incorporate it. Keep adding clay until the mixture is smooth and about the consistency of yogurt. Blend in the essential oil.

Store in a tightly capped container in the shower for up to 1 week.

To Use: Wet your hair. Starting at roots, massage a handful of the clay mixture into hair and work down to the roots. Repeat until all hair is coated. Leave for 5 to 20 minutes—but do not let dry! Rinse out with warm water.

Optional: Rinse with 1 cup reserved herb-vinegar tea.

Note: Bentonite clay is most effective if it doesn't come in contact with metal prior to use. Mix the ingredients in a wood, plastic, or glass bowl for best results, though I haven't found that this makes much of a difference for hair products. I use an old mini–food processor with a plastic dough blade that I found at a thrift shop.

Clay Hair Detox

1 cup brewed, strained herbal tea (choose Herbal Hair Detox for Blonde Hair on page 198 or Herbal Hair Detox for Brown or Black Hair on page 199, depending on your hair color) or water

½ cup apple cider vinegar

Approximately ¾ cup bentonite or redmond clay

5 drops lavender essential oil (optional)

5 drops rosemary essential oil (optional)

Pour the tea and vinegar in a blender. (Alternatively, you can whisk together the ingredients in a nonmetal bowl.) Add the clay 1 tablespoon at a time while blending to incorporate it. Keep adding clay until the mixture is smooth and about the consistency of yogurt. Blend in the essential oils (if using).

Store in a tightly capped container in the shower for up to 1 week.

To Use: Wet your hair. Starting at roots, massage a handful of the clay mixture into hair and work down to the roots. Repeat until all hair is coated. Leave for 5 to 20 minutes—but do not let dry! Rinse out with warm water.

Optional: Rinse your hair with 1 cup herb-vinegar tea.

Note: Bentonite clay is most effective if it doesn't come in contact with metal prior to use. Mix with wood, plastic, or glass for best results, though I haven't found that this makes much of a difference for hair products. I use an old mini–food processor with a plastic dough blade that I found at a thrift shop.

Light Hair Color Rinse

½ cup fresh lemon juice

2 cups strong chamomile tea

2 cups strong calendula tea (optional, for more golden tones)

Combine the lemon juice, chamomile tea, and (if using) the calendula tea in a spray or other small bottle and shake well. Spray onto or pour into the hair and brush through to get even. This works best when applied to hair directly before sun exposure and left in for 1 to 2 hours before being rinsed out. This mixture may be used several times a week until desired color is reached. Shake well before each use.

You can also use this as a rinse at the end of a shower. Rinse lightly with water afterward. This will not have an overnight dramatic effect, though I definitely noticed a difference after putting it in my hair and gardening in the sun for a few hours.

Red Hair Color Rinse (herbs for red hair)

The herbs in the recipe below will create a red/dark strawberry blonde tint in lighter hair and an auburn tint in darker hair. The effects are cumulative, so extended use over time will create a more vibrant red. If you want continual red hair, make this rinse part of your regular hair care routine.

½ cup fresh calendula flowers or fresh marigold petals from your garden

2 tablespoons hibiscus petals (available from Mountain Rose Herbs)

In a small saucepan, bring to a boil 2 cups water and add the flowers and petals. Reduce the heat and simmer for at least 30 minutes. Remove from the heat and let cool.

Pour through a strainer into a jar or bottle. Discard the solids. Store the rinse in the jar or bottle in the refrigerator for up to a week. Use as a final hair rinse at the end of each shower. Dry your hair in the sun if possible. Repeat daily until the desired shade is achieved and then every few days to maintain.

Brown Hair Color Rinse

2 cups water
¼ cup dried nettle leaf
¼ cup dried rosemary
¼ cup dried sage

In a small saucepan, bring water to a boil and add the herbs. Reduce the heat and simmer for at least 30 minutes, or until water is very dark. Remove from heat and let cool.

Pour through a strainer into a jar or bottle. Discard the solids. Store the rinse in the jar or bottle in the refrigerator for up to a week. Spray onto or brush into your hair about an hour before showering each day; then shampoo as normal. This mixture can also be used as a rinse and left on at the end of each shower. Repeat daily until the desired shade is achieved. It has a cumulative effect and you probably won't notice much difference the first few days. The herbs in this mix are also great for getting rid of dandruff and for increasing hair growth.

Gelatin Hair Restoration Treatment

1 tablespoon gelatin powder
1 teaspoon apple cider vinegar
1 teaspoon honey

Place the gelatin powder in a small bowl, add ½ cup cool water, and stir until dissolved. Add ½ cup warm to hot water, the vinegar, and the honey to create a thick gel. Pour on your hair and massage through your hair and scalp. Leave on for at least 5 minutes and rinse with hot water. Shampoo as usual.

Coconut Oil Hair Treatment

4 tablespoons unrefined coconut oil, melted

1 tablespoon honey

Mix together the oil and honey. Massage it through your hair. Leave it on for at least 20 minutes and then wash normally.

Dry Shampoo for Light Hair

¼ cup arrowroot powder or organic cornstarch

5 drops essential oil of choice

Place the arrowroot in a small glass bowl, add the essential oil, and stir together to combine. Store the mixture in a small glass jar or repurposed powder container.

Using an old makeup brush, apply the mixture to the roots or oily parts of your hair. Using the brush is optional, but it removes the need to comb through as much and is better for styled hair. If you don't use the brush, comb the powder through your hair and style as usual.

Dry Shampoo for Dark Hair

2 tablespoons arrowroot/cornstarch

2 tablespoons cocoa powder

5 drops essential oil of choice

In a small glass bowl, stir together the arrowroot and cocoa powder. Add the essential oil and mix with a spoon until well incorporated. Store the mixture in a small glass jar or repurposed powder container.

Using an old makeup brush, apply the mixture to the roots or oily parts of your hair. Using with the brush is optional, but it removes the need to comb through as much and is better for styled hair. If you don't use the brush, comb the powder through your hair and style as usual.

DIY Wet/Dry Spray Shampoo for Light or Dark Hair

1/4 cup arrowroot or cornstarch

1/4 cup vodka, rubbing alcohol, or witch hazel

Essential oil or a spritz of your favorite perfume to scent

Mix the arrowroot, vodka, essential oil, and 1 cup warm water in a small spray bottle and shake well. Spray on roots or oily parts of hair. Let dry and style as usual. Shake well before each use. Store in a spray bottle at room temperature for up to 2 months.

Soap Nuts Shampoo

Finding a natural shampoo that works for your hair type can be difficult. Soap nuts can be used to make a really easy natural shampoo or body wash that is soothing to eczema or psoriasis. Soap nuts shampoo is also incredibly inexpensive to make and completely natural. Tip: If you make a full batch, store in ice cube trays and freeze for individual-use sizes or store in a peri-bottle in the refrigerator and just take out when you shower. If you aren't up for making it and want a more involved (but still natural) solution, you can purchase a natural store-bought soap nuts shampoo.

5 soap nuts
5 drops lavender essential oil

Bring to a boil in a medium saucepan 2 cups water. Place the soap nuts in a small muslin bag and add to the saucepan. Reduce the heat and simmer for 20 minutes. Add 1 cup water and return to a simmer for 10 more minutes. Remove from the heat and let cool. Add the lavender essential oil.

Remove the bag from the saucepan and squeeze it out into the pan until it suds. Rinse the bag with cool water and squeeze it into the pan again.

Store in a tightly capped glass jar in the refrigerator until ready to use.

To Use: Massage a small amount into hair, and let sit for 5 minutes. Rinse well.

Sea Salt Texturizing Hair Spray

1 cup hot water (not boiling), strong chamomile tea
(if you want to lighten hair), or black tea
(if you want to darken your hair)

2 tablespoons Epsom salts, plus more if extra texture is desired

1/2 teaspoon Himalayan sea salt (optional but adds stiffness)

1 teaspoon aloe vera gel

1/2 teaspoon natural conditioner of choice (optional; don't use if you have fine or oily hair)

A few drops lavender or citrus essential oil or a spritz of your favorite perfume to scent (optional)

1 teaspoon fresh lemon juice + 1 teaspoon vodka or food-grade alcohol, if you want to lighten hair
(the lemon juice lightens and the alcohol preserves it)

Get a glass spray bottle that holds at least 10 ounces.

Pour the hot water in the spray bottle and add the Epsom salts, sea salt (if using), aloe vera gel, conditioner (if using), essential oil (if using) and lemon juice/vodka (if using). Cap tightly and shake until the Epsom salts are dissolved, 1 to 2 minutes. Store in the refrigerator if using lemon juice or tea base or at room temperature if you aren't. The spray will last up to 2 months.

To Use: Spray on damp hair and scrunch with a towel to dry for loose beach waves. Alternatively, spray on dry hair and on roots for volume and texture without the waves.

If your hair is straight and thin and you want all-day waves: Wash your hair the night before and spray hair while still damp. Then either French braid into pigtails or wrap in a tight scrunched bun on top of your head, and leave overnight. By morning, your hair should be dry. Spritz with a little more spray and take out the braid/bun. Voilà: all-day beach waves. Spray with additional spray and scrunch if you want more stiffness.

Hair Spray

1½ cups filtered water

2 tablespoons sugar (must be white)

1 tablespoon spiced rum or vodka (I prefer spiced rum for the scent)

10 to 15 drops essential oil of choice

In a small saucepan, bring the water to a boil and dissolve sugar in it. Remove from the heat and let cool to room temperature. Add the rum and essential oil. Use as a regular hair spray. Store in an airtight spray bottle and it will last indefinitely.

Note: Adjust the sugar up or down for more or less stiffness and hold (more sugar = stronger hold), but don't add too much or your hair will feel sticky. For a texturizing spray, I've had some luck reducing the sugar by half and adding 1 tablespoon Epsom salts.

Silky Smooth Detangling Spray

This detangling spray leaves hair shiny without weighing it down or making it oily.

12-ounce or larger spray bottle

1½ cups distilled water

3 tablespoons marshmallow root

2 tablespoons natural conditioner of choice

5 drops rosemary essential oil (optional)

In a small saucepan, bring to a boil the water and marshmallow root. Reduce the heat and let simmer for 20 to 30 minutes. Let cool slightly.

Pour through a strainer into a small glass bowl. Discard the solids. While still warm, pour into a 12-ounce spray bottle and add the conditioner and essential oil (if using). Cap tightly and shake well until mixed.

Store at room temperature for up to one month (this is as long as I've tested its shelf life).

Beard Oil

½ ounce argan oil
¼ ounce jojoba oil
¼ ounce sweet almond oil
7 drops lavender essential oil
5 drops rosemary essential oil
3 drops cedarwood essential oil

Combine all the ingredients in a 1-ounce amber glass bottle with a dropper. Cap tightly and gently swirl to incorporate.

To use: Depending on beard length, apply 3 to 5 drops to beard and rub through with fingertips. (Longer beards will require more drops but remember, a little goes a long way, so increase amount by one drop at a time.) When all the oil has been applied, use fingertips to massage oil down into the beard all the way to the skin. Use a small comb to smooth down the beard. For best results, apply daily to freshly washed beard that has been toweled dry.

Natural Hair Growth Oil

¼ cup castor oil
1 teaspoon black cumin seed oil
½ teaspoon rosemary-infused oil (see page 50)
15 drops lavender essential oil (optional)

Combine all the ingredients in a dark glass bottle. Cap tightly and gently swirl to incorporate.

To use, moisten hair and massage 10 to 30 drops (or ½ to 1 teaspoon) into the scalp. Leave on for at least 1 hour or up to overnight, then shampoo. I recommend sleeping with a towel on the pillow to avoid oil stains. I use this once a week to increase hair growth.

Note: Test the oils on a small part of the inner arm before using on the entire scalp and do not use if it causes any reaction or sensitivity. Black cumin seed oil can irritate the skin for a small percentage of people with sensitive skin.

Natural Bar Shave Soap

This is an easy way to modify a regular bar soap to make it more shave-friendly. It is a little time consuming, but these bar soaps last a long time and are great for using shave mugs if the men in your life happen to use shave mugs and brushes.

    1 bar of natural handcrafted soap (store-bought substitutes won't work)
    1 tablespoon olive or almond oil or aloe vera gel
    1 to 2 tablespoons white cosmetic, French green, or kaolin clay

Grate the soap and place in a small saucepan over low heat. Add the oil and melt. It will take at least five minutes, so be patient and stir often.

Once melted, stir in the clay (this makes a richer lather and is great for the skin).

Pour into molds (I use cardboard) or old mugs and let set for several days until it rehardens. Will last months and will cure more over time, making it longer lasting.

Bentonite Detox Bath

I often add about ¼ cup of bentonite clay to a bath for a relaxing detox bath that softens skin.

My Favorite Magnesium Bath

1 to 2 cups Epsom salt or magnesium chloride flakes
½ cup Himalayan or sea salt
½ teaspoon pure vanilla extract
10 to 15 drops essential oil of choice (I love lavender and mint)

Mix the Epsom salt and Himalayan salt and then sprinkle with the vanilla and essential oil. Add to a warm bath and soak for 20 to 30 minutes.

Lavender Melaleuca Deodorant Bar

Try making your own deodorant if you haven't already. My homemade versions work just as well—and I can save money and avoid chemicals.

- ½ cup unrefined coconut oil
- ½ cup shea, cocoa, or mango butter (or an equal mix of each)
- ½ cup plus 1 teaspoon beeswax
- 3 tablespoons baking soda (replace with arrowroot or cornstarch if you have sensitive skin)
- ½ cup arrowroot powder
- 20 drops lavender essential oil
- ~~5~~ drops melaleuca essential oil

10   *20 drops Purify (RMO)*

Place the coconut oil, shea butter, and beeswax in a quart-size mason jar and cap loosely. Place the jar in a small saucepan with 1 inch water and bring to a boil until melted and smooth. (You can just designate this jar for this type of project and not even need to wash it out.)

Remove from the heat and add the baking soda, arrowroot, and essential oils. Gently stir by hand until all are incorporated.

If you're making these into bars, pour into muffin tins or other molds while still liquid. If you're putting into an old deodorant container to use like stick deodorant, let the mixture harden for about 15 to 20 minutes at room temperature. When it is about the consistency of peanut butter, scoop the deodorant into the container and pack down to fill. Then leave the cap off overnight to completely harden prior to using.

So far I don't like this recipe as well as the one I usually use. So much oil & wax, I don't feel dry

Made 1/21/2019
3   2.5 oz deo tubes
1   15 ml " "
½ brown jar

Prefer:
½ c. coconut oil
¼ c arrowroot
2 T baking soda
25 drops lavender
25 drops purification
10 drops thieves

more like recipe → paper

Lemon-Coconut Spreadable Deodorant

This deodorant won't hold up well as a bar or in a deodorant container, but it is a great simple recipe that is really fast to make.

- ½ cup unrefined coconut oil
- ¼ cup arrowroot powder
- 2 tablespoons baking soda (can be omitted for anyone with sensitive skin)
- 20 drops lemon or other skin-safe essential oil (optional)

In a small saucepan over low heat, melt the oil. Stir in arrowroot, baking soda, and (if using) the essential oil. Pour into a small glass jar and let cool until hardened.

To use: Rub a pea-size amount into each armpit.

Magnesium-Infused Spray Deodorant

Some people with sensitive skin react to deodorants containing baking soda. An armpit detox can help (Google "Wellness Mama Armpit Detox" to find it), but a magnesium-based deodorant is another great alternative.

- 4 ounces magnesium oil
- 10 drops essential oil of choice (optional)

Pour into a 5-ounce glass spray bottle. Cap tightly and shake gently to combine. Use as a spray deodorant.

Note: Because of the mineral content in the magnesium oil, it can sting when sprayed on skin after shaving.

Detoxification Oil-Pulling Blend

½ cup sesame oil

½ cup sunflower or coconut oil

10 drops peppermint essential oil

2 drops clove essential oil

Place all the ingredients in a small glass jar, cap tightly, and shake to mix. Swish 1 tablespoon in the mouth for 20 minutes. Spit the oil into the trash can (not into the sink drain!) and rinse mouth well. Brush as normal. Store at room temperature for up to 2 months.

Cinna-Mint Oil-Pulling Chews

½ cup unrefined coconut oil

10 drops cinnamon essential oil

5 drops peppermint essential oil

In a small saucepan over low heat, melt the oil. Stir in essential oils until combined. Carefully pour into silicone bite-size candy molds and place in the freezer. Freeze for 1 hour. Remove and pop out of the molds. Store in a small glass jar in the refrigerator until ready to use. For use, place one "chew" in the mouth. Chew until melted and swish for 20 minutes. Spit the oil into the trash can (not into the sink drain!) and rinse mouth well. Brush as usual.

Pure Peppermint Homemade Toothpaste

For clean, smooth teeth, use baking soda as a part of a simple homemade toothpaste that is not too abrasive.

> 1/2 cup calcium carbonate powder
> 1 tablespoon baking soda
> 1/4 cup xylitol powder (optional; keeps the toothpaste from tasting bitter)
> About 1/2 cup unrefined coconut oil or 1/4 cup almond oil
> 10 drops peppermint essential oil (optional)

In a small glass bowl, mix together the calcium carbonate, baking soda, and (if using) the xylitol. Add the oil a little at a time, stirring, until you get desired paste consistency. Mix in the essential oil (if using).

Store in a tightly capped small glass jar for up to 6 months.

To use, either dip clean toothbrush into it, or use a Popsicle stick or spoon to put on toothbrush. (We use separate jars for each family member.)

Four-Ingredient Whitening Toothpaste

This simple whitening toothpaste is very easy to make and it tastes great! I find that my kids prefer this recipe.

> 1/4 cup calcium carbonate powder
> 3 tablespoons finely ground xylitol
> 1/4 cup sesame oil
> 10 drops peppermint, cinnamon, or clove essential oil (optional)

In a small glass bowl, mix together the calcium carbonate, xylitol, and oil. Stir in the essential oil (if using). Store in a tightly capped small glass jar for up to 2 months. Use just like a regular toothpaste.

Cinnamon and Clove Clay Tooth Powder

4 tablespoons bentonite clay

3 tablespoons calcium carbonate powder

1 tablespoon baking soda (optional)

1 tablespoon ground cinnamon or 10 drops cinnamon essential oil (optional)

½ teaspoon ground cloves or 3 drops clove essential oil (optional)

1 tablespoon finely ground xylitol powder, or more to taste

In a small glass bowl, mix together the clay, calcium carbonate, baking soda (if using), cinnamon (if using), cloves, and xylitol. Store in a tightly capped glass jar. (We use separate jars for each family member.) This recipe makes about ¾ cup of tooth powder, which lasts us for months. You can adjust the recipe up or down.

You can customize the powder to your taste and all the spices are optional. Bentonite or baking soda can work alone or together as a tooth powder. You could also add more cloves and cinnamon for an even more concentrated powder. This type of cinnamon has a higher concentration of beneficial oils and tastes sweeter.

Charcoal Whitening Tooth Powder

½ cup activated charcoal

1 teaspoon finely ground xylitol

10 drops peppermint essential oil

In a small glass bowl, mix together the charcoal and xylitol. Stir in the essential oil until well incorporated. Store in a tightly capped small glass jar for up to 6 months.

To use, dip toothbrush into the mixture and brush as usual. (We use separate jars for each family member.) Rinse well and swish with clean water until all charcoal residue is gone.

Herbal Mouthwash

2 tablespoons dried peppermint

2 tablespoons dried plantain leaf

1 tablespoon dried rosemary

1 teaspoon whole or ground cloves

Boiling water

1 cup vodka

15 drops cinnamon or peppermint essential oil, or more to taste (optional)

Place the peppermint, plantain leaf, rosemary, and cloves in a pint-size mason jar. Pour in just enough boiling water to dampen. (This helps release the properties of the herbs.) Pour in the vodka, cap tightly, and let rest in a cool, dark place for 2 to 3 weeks, shaking daily.

Pour through a strainer into a small glass jar or tincture vials. Discard the solids. Add the essential oil (if using), cap tightly, and shake well. Store on the bathroom counter with a small cup or glass nearby.

To use: For each use, mix a mouthful of water with about 40 drops of the tincture and swish well for 30 seconds. For extra cleansing, add 40 drops of the tincture to a half-and-half mixture of hydrogen peroxide and water instead of plain water and swish for 30 seconds.

Babies are the most susceptible to harmful chemicals in personal care and other products, so homemade alternatives are the way to go. Of course, it is important to be gentle and use caution on baby skin, and even some safe natural remedies should not be used on baby, including most essential oils. And babies under age two should not ingest honey. Check with a pediatrician or doctor before using any herb or remedy on baby, even externally.

Natural Diaper Cream

¼ cup shea butter

¼ cup unrefined coconut oil

1 tablespoon beeswax pastilles

2 tablespoons fermented cod liver oil

2 tablespoons zinc oxide powder

1 tablespoon bentonite clay

A few drops of chamomile essential oil (optional)

In a double boiler over low heat, melt the shea butter, coconut oil, and beeswax. (I keep a double boiler just for making beauty products since it is difficult to clean dishes after making anything with beeswax or zinc oxide.)

Remove from the heat and add the cod liver oil, zinc oxide, clay, and (if using) essential oil. Stir carefully as it starts to cool. I recommend using a Popsicle stick or disposable straw to stir so it can be discarded since it is difficult to get the mixture off dishes.

Pour into a small glass jar, stirring occasionally as it cools. Store in a cool, dry place for up to 3 months.

Use as needed for diaper rash.

Vitamin-Rich Baby Oil

1 cup organic olive or apricot kernel oil (softer scent and great for sensitive skin)
2 tablespoons dried calendula flowers
2 tablespoons dried chamomile flowers

There are two ways to make this recipe.

The fast way: In a double boiler over medium-high heat, warm the oil. Add the flowers, reduce the heat to medium-low, and let simmer until oil has started to turn yellow and smells of chamomile and calendula, at least 1 hour. Check the water level in the double boiler often to make sure it hasn't gotten too hot or evaporated off.

Pour through a strainer into a small glass jar. Discard the solids. Cap tightly and store in a cool, dark place. Use as you would regular baby oil.

The slower, more concentrated way: Place the flowers in a small glass jar and pour the oil over them. Cap tightly and let rest in a cool, dark place for 6 to 8 weeks, shaking daily. This will make a gorgeous light orange oil that is great for baby or adult skin. It is soothing on eczema or skin irritation and calming to baby.

Natural Baby Powder

1 teaspoon dried chamomile or calendula flowers or 5 drops of chamomile essential oil
½ cup arrowroot powder

Place the flowers in a mini–food processor and process till powdered. Remove to a small glass bowl and mix in the arrowroot. Store in a small glass jar or sugar shaker for easy use. Use as you would regular baby powder.

DIY Baby Wipes

Roll of heavy-duty paper towels (I use Bounty for wipes; cheap paper towels do not work for wipes . . . I've tried)

Rubbermaid #6 or #8 container (old wipes container, plastic coffee container, or gallon-size plastic ice cream bucket also work)

1¾ cups boiled water, cooled but still warm (tap water can be used if you use the wipes in less than a week like we do)

1 tablespoon aloe vera gel

1 tablespoon pure witch hazel extract

1 tablespoon liquid castile soap, such as Dr. Bronner's

10 drops grapefruit seed extract or 2 capsules of vitamin E (optional)

1 teaspoon olive or almond oil (optional)

Essential oils of choice (I use 6 drops each of orange and lavender) (optional)

Using a sharp knife, cut the roll of paper towels in half horizontally. Place the wipes cut side down in the container. (If using an old wipes container, accordion-fold the wipes into the container.)

In a quart-size mason jar, stir together the water, aloe vera gel, witch hazel, castile soap, grapefruit seed extract, and oil. Stir in the essential oils (if using).

Pour the mixture over the paper towels in container and let absorb, 5 to 10 minutes. Flip the container over to make sure wipes are well soaked.

Pull out the cardboard roll from the inside of the paper towels. This should also pull the innermost wipe out and get them started for you.

Use as you would regular wipes, and smile, knowing you are not causing your beautiful child any future health problems!

Note: If your child has extremely sensitive skin, you may need to leave out the essential oils or use calendula or chamomile instead.

Reusable Homemade Wipes

Wipes don't have to be disposable; you can make reusable ones too. Just cut up old clean receiving blankets and T-shirts into 8 × 8-inch squares. Fold them into old wipes containers and pour the DIY Baby Wipes (page 219) mixture onto them. The wipes mixture may also be stored in a glass spray bottle. To use, spray some of the mixture on your cloth wipe. These reusable wipes are an even cheaper option, and I try using them all the time.

Chamomile Tincture for Teething

½ to 1 cup dried chamomile flowers
Boiling water
1½ to 1¾ cups vodka or rum

Place the flowers in a quart-size glass jar and pour in just enough boiling water to cover (you may have to stir). Fill the rest of the jar with the vodka and cap tightly. Let rest in a cool, dark place for 4 to 6 weeks, shaking daily. This will make a strong tincture!

Pour through a strainer into small glass jars or tincture vials. Discard the solids. Cap tightly and store at room temperature in a cool, dark place.

Chamomile-Calendula Baby Salve (External Use Only)

1 cup chamomile and calendula–infused oil (see page 50)

⅓ cup beeswax pastilles

3 drops lavender essential oil

In a double boiler over low heat, melt the oil and beeswax. Remove from the heat and stir in lavender essential oil (if using) Quickly pour into small jars or tins and let cool and harden completely. Use as needed on skin. Store at room temperature for up to 3 years. (At temperatures above 85°F, the salve will melt.)

Natural Cleaning Recipes

Citrus-Fresh All-Purpose Cleaner

I use this cleaner just about everywhere in my home: on floors and patio furniture and in trash cans and the bathroom, to name a few. It is very easy to make and considerably less expensive than other natural cleaners. Give it a try and attack those tough stains!

1 teaspoon borax

½ teaspoon washing soda

1 teaspoon liquid castile soap

2 cups distilled water or boiling water, cooled but still warm

4 drops lemon essential oil

10 drops orange essential oil

Place borax, washing soda, and castile soap in a 16-ounce or larger glass spray bottle. Add the water and essential oils, cap tightly, and shake well.

Use as needed. I use as a bathroom cleaner, floor pretreater (test a small area first on wood floors), and all-purpose kitchen cleaner and on toys to disinfect. Will last 6 months at room temperature.

laundry

Fifteen years ago, I first considered the idea of homemade laundry detergent after watching a friend's mom make hers, and I've been experimenting with recipes ever since. My laundry detergent recipes are an easy switch from their store-bought counterparts. They're just as effective and much less expensive. Plus, they help you avoid the harsh chemicals, fragrances, colors, and additives in many regular detergents.

I offer both a powder and a liquid recipe. The powder is much faster to make and requires much less room to store, but the liquid is more effective for stain treating. The liquid also seems a better option for those with hard water. I currently use the powdered detergent and Natural Stain Remover Spray (page 225). Just choose the option that works best for you.

Fresh Lemon-Powdered Laundry Detergent

- 1 bar coconut-based or castile soap
- 1 cup washing soda
- 1 cup borax (or substitute 1 additional cup washing soda)
- 20 drops lemon essential oil (optional)
- 20 drops lime essential oil (optional)

Using a hand grater, grate the soap into fine particles so that it will dissolve easily. Place in a large bowl. Add the washing soda and borax and mix (wear gloves or use a spoon as these can be drying if they come into direct contact with skin). Add the essential oils (if using) and stir.

Store in a pint-size mason jar.

To use, add 1 to 2 tablespoons per load. Add 1 tablespoon Homemade Oxygen Booster (page 227) if needed. I like to add the booster to white loads.

Note: Do you have a high-efficiency (HE) washing machine? I don't, but I've heard from dozens of my blog readers who do, and they've used this detergent in an HE washer with no problems. The main concern with an HE washer is that it tends to create too many suds, which is why the manufacturers suggest using low-suds detergents. This recipe should be safe for HE, but check with the manufacturer's instructions that came with your machine to make sure.

Optional Add-Ins: I've also experimented with adding OxiClean or a homemade booster to this recipe. I've found that they don't do much good when mixed into the recipe but can be great when added to especially dirty loads of laundry along with the homemade soap.

Unscented Liquid Laundry Detergent

⅓ cup borax
⅓ cup washing soda
⅓ cup Dr. Bronner's Sal Suds

Pour the borax and washing soda into a jug or container. Add 3 cups hot water and stir until they dissolve. Add the suds and 1 more cup hot water and gently stir.

To use, add ¼ cup per load. For stain treatment, pour some directly on stain immediately before washing.

What About Those Really Tough Stains?

When I encounter stains that don't respond to the methods above, I use stronger products that are still natural. My favorites are Branch Basics (find it here: WellnessMama.com/go/branch-basics), which is completely natural, inert, and plant based, and Dr. Bronner's Sal Suds, which gets an A rating from the Environmental Working Group and is an amazing all-purpose natural cleaner. It can be applied directly to really tough stains in a pinch, though I prefer to make a natural stain spray. It's nontoxic, takes just a couple minutes to make, and can be kept by the washing machine for easy use.

Natural Stain Remover Spray

¼ cup Dr. Bronner's Sal Suds (regular Dr. Bronner's Liquid Castile Soap will not work the same way in this recipe) or Branch Basics Concentrate

Pour 1¾ cups water into a 16-ounce spray bottle. Add the suds, cap tightly, and swirl gently to combine. Spray on tough stains before laundering.

Other Natural Laundry Strategies

I take my job as home manager very seriously, and I like to have my laundry situation in control so I can take care of other things more efficiently. Here are some additional strategies that really work and save time:

Laundry Booster

Add 1 tablespoon Branch Basics or Dr. Bronner's Sal Suds to a load of laundry as a natural stain-removing booster.

Dryer Static Eliminator

Natural dryer sheets are a great way to remove static, and they can be reused.

1 cup white vinegar
25 to 30 drops essential oils of choice (I like geranium, citrus, lavender, and mint or a mixture)
24 cloth baby wipes or old scraps of clean cloth cut into 8-inch squares
Wide-mouthed mason jar

Mix together the vinegar with the essential oils of choice in a bowl or jar.

Fold the wipes and place in your storage jar. Slowly pour in the vinegar–essential oil mixture. You want to moisten, not saturate, the cloths. Extra mixture can be stored in a capped bottle.

To use, add 1 wipe per dryer load to freshen laundry and reduce static. The vinegar smell will evaporate during drying and the essential oil scent will remain.

Wool Dryer Balls

Wool dryer balls help remove static and also shorten the time it takes to dry a load of laundry. I couldn't believe it took me so long to try them, and I won't ever go back. The mixture of natural dryer sheets and dryer balls has been the perfect solution for me. You can often find these at local health food stores or grocery stores and they are also available online.

Homemade Oxygen Booster

Of all the stain removers out there, OxiClean is the most natural option that I've found, but it is also one of the most expensive. After seeing recipes for a homemade stain-removing booster, I tested my own versions until I found one that works! From my own "scientific" testing (on my kids' laundry), it seems to be as effective as the store-bought stuff. It's also really easy and inexpensive to make! Please note that this is best made fresh and not stored. I keep the hydrogen peroxide and washing soda in my laundry area and mix small batches to use as needed.

2 tablespoons water
1 tablespoon hydrogen peroxide
1 tablespoon washing soda

Combine all ingredients in a glass mixing cup as needed to use them. Don't make more than you're going to use for the day's laundry because the mixture loses effectiveness if stored.

To use, spray on stains to pretreat or add the entire mixture to a load of laundry, fill the washing machine with water, and let soak for 30 minutes before washing.

Your laundry space is one of the hardest working areas in your home—and often the tiniest. By adopting some of these strategies, you create a certain tranquillity in your house and bring peace to an often-dreaded chore.

Citrus-Blend Dishwasher Detergent

1 cup borax
1 cup washing soda
$\frac{1}{2}$ cup citric acid
$\frac{1}{2}$ cup salt
40 drops lemon essential oil
20 drops orange essential oil

Mix together all the ingredients in a quart-size mason jar. Use as you would any commercial dishwasher powder.

Lemon-Rosemary Scouring Powder

Nasty tubs or floors? This homemade scouring powder works really well.

1 cup baking soda
$\frac{1}{2}$ cup salt (not iodized)
$\frac{1}{2}$ cup washing soda
25 drops lemon essential oil (for scent)
10 drops rosemary essential oil (for killing bacteria)

Mix together all the ingredients in a pint-size mason jar and cap tightly. If you want to make a shaker, using a sharp serrated knife, carefully poke some holes in the top of a metal mason jar lid. Or, save the top of a Parmesan cheese container and screw it onto the mason jar to make a shaker top!

To use, lightly wet the affected surface with water or, for really bad messes, with undiluted white vinegar. Sprinkle on the scouring powder and let sit for 5 minutes. Scrub with a sturdy brush until clean. Rinse with water or, if needed, vinegar.

Lemon-Shine Glass Cleaner

1 tablespoon white vinegar
10 drops lemon essential oil

Pour 1 cup water into an 8-ounce or larger glass spray bottle and add the vinegar and essential oil. Cap tightly and shake to mix. Use as needed to clean windows. I like to use a microfiber cloth with this cleaner.

Note: If you have always used commercial window cleaner in the past, mix a couple drops liquid castile soap or natural liquid dish soap in with this cleaner the first time you use it—it will help remove any detergent residue from the glass.

REFERENCES

Chapter One

Arnold, L. E., N. Lofthouse, and E. Hurt, "Artificial Food Colors and Attention-Deficit/Hyperactivity Symptoms: Conclusions to Dye For," *Neurotherapeutics* 9(3) (July 2012): 599–609.

"Artificial Sweetener May Disrupt Body's Ability to Count Calories, According to New Study," June 30, 2004, available at https://www.sciencedaily.com/releases/2004/06/040630081825.htm.

"Artificial Sweeteners Linked to Weight Gain," February 11, 2008, available at https://www.sciencedaily.com/releases/2008/02/080210183902.htm.

Bellisle, F., and A. Drewnowski, "Intense Sweeteners, Energy Intake and the Control of Body Weight," February 7, 2007, available at https://www.nature.com/articles/1602649.

Benachour, N., and G. E. Seralini, "Glyphosate Formulations Induce Apoptosis and Necrosis in Human Umbilical, Embryonic, and Placental Cells," *Chemical Research in Toxicology* 22 (1) (2009): 97–105.

Benigni, R., C. Bossa, and O. Tcheremenskaia, "Nongenotoxic Carcinogenicity of Chemicals: Mechanisms of Action and Early Recognition Through a New Set of Structural Alerts," *Chemical Reviews* 113 (5) (2013): 2940–2957.

Brown, R. J., and K. I. Rother, "Non-nutritive Sweeteners and Their Role in the Gastrointestinal Tract," *The Journal of Clinical Endocrinology & Metabolism* 97 (8) (August 2012): 2597–2605.

Cakmak, et. al., "Residential Exposure to Volatile Organic Compounds and Lung Function: Results from a Population-Based Cross-sectional Survey," *Environmental Pollution* 194 (November 2014): 141–151.

Cashman, A. L., and E. M. Warshaw, "Parabens: A Review of Epidemiology, Structure, Allergenicity, and Hormonal Properties," *Dermatitis* 16(2) (June 2005): 57–6; quiz 55–6.

Centers for Disease Control and Prevention, Department of Health and Human Services, National Center for Environmental Health. Fourth National Report on Human Exposure to Environmental Chemicals, 2009.

Centers for Disease Control Report, "National Report on Human Exposure to Environmental Chemicals," 2001, available at https://www.cdc.gov/exposurereport/index.html.

Chin, et. al., "Levels and Sources of Volatile Organic Compounds in Homes of Children with Asthma," *Indoor Air* 24(4) (August 2014): 403–415.

Curtis, L, "Toxicity of Fragrances [Letter]," *Environmental Health Perspectives* 112 (2004): A461.

Gammon, C., "Weed-Whacking Herbicide Proves Deadly to Human Cells," June 23, 2009, available at https://www.scientificamerican.com/article/weed-whacking-herbicide-p/.

Goettlich, Paul, "What are Endocrine Disruptors?," 2001.

Green, E., and C. Murphy, "Altered Processing of Sweet Taste in the Brain of Diet Soda Drinkers," *Physiology & Behavior* 107 (4) (November 5, 2012): 560–7.

Greim, H., D. Saltmiras, V. Mostert, and C. Strupp, "Evaluation of Carcinogenic Potential of the Herbicide Glyphosate, Drawing on Tumor Incidence Data from Fourteen Chronic Carcinogenicity Rodent Studies," *Critical Reviews in Toxicology* 45 (3) (2015): 185–208.

Harvey, P. W., and P. Darbre, "Endocrine Disrupters and Human Health: Could Oestrogenic Chemicals in Body Care Cosmetics Adversely Affect Breast Cancer Incidence in Women?," *Journal of Applied Toxicology* 24 (3) (May–June 2004): 167–76.

Heydens, W. F., C. E. Healy, K. J. Hotz, L. D. Kier, M. A. Martens, A. G. E. Wilson, et al., "Genotoxic Potential of Glyphosate Formulations: Mode-of-Action Investigations," *Journal of Agricultural and Food Chemistry* 5 6 (4) (2008): 1517–1523.

Kresser, C., K. Huffman, D. M. S. Hamilton-Gibbs, R. Snoopy Storey, March 22, 2017, "The Unbiased Truth About Artificial Sweeteners," available at https://chriskresser.com/the-unbiased-truth-about-artificial -sweeteners/.

Lordon, J. F., and A. Claude, "Behavioral and Endocrinological Effects of Single Injections of Monosodium Glutamate in the Mouse," *Neurobehavioral Toxicology and Teratology* 8.5 (1986): 509–19. Print.

Mooney, C., "In a Surprising Study, Scientists Say Everyday Chemicals Now Rival Cars as a Source of Air Pollution," *The Washington Post*, February, 15, 2008, available at https://www.washingtonpost.com/ news/energy-environment/wp/2018/02/15/in-a-surprising-study-scientists-say-everyday-chemicals -now-rival-cars-as-a-source-of-air-pollution/?noredirect=on&utm_term=.2f67cf070fde.

Mukund, R., T. J. Kelly, and C. W. Spicer, "Source Attribution of Ambient Air Toxic and Other VOCs in Columbus, Ohio," *Atmospheric Environment* 30 (20) (1996): 3457–3470.

"Non-nutritive Sweeteners Can Increase Insulin Resistance in Those Who Are Obese," December 3, 2016, available at http://www.diabetesincontrol.com/non-nutritive-sweeteners-can-increase-insulin -resistance-in-those-who-are-obese/.

Potera, C., "Indoor Air Quality: Scented Products Emit a Bouquet of VOCs," *Environmental Health Perspectives* 119(1) (January 2011): A16.

"The Problem with Plastics—Yale Ecology Center Plastic Task Force Report," Berkeley, CA, 1996, available at https://ecologycenter.org/wp-content/uploads/2013/04/PTF_1996.pdf.

Renwick, A. G., and S. V. Molinary, "Sweet-Taste Receptors, Low-Energy Sweeteners, Glucose Absorption and Insulin Release," *British Journal of Nutrition,* July 12, 2010.

Rowe, K. S., and K. J. Rowe, "Synthetic Food Coloring and Behavior: A Dose Response Effect in a Double-Blind, Placebo-Controlled, Repeated-Measures Study," *The Journal of Pediatric*s Vol. 125 (November 1994).

Rudenga, K. J., and D. M. Small, "Amygdala Response to Sucrose Consumption Is Inversely Related to Artificial Sweetener Use," *Appetite* 58 (2) (April 2012): 504–7.

Salvito, D. T., R. J. Senna, and T. W. Federle, "A Framework for Prioritizing Fragrance Materials for Aquatic Risk Assessment," *Environmental Toxicology and Chemistry* 21(6) (2002): 1301–1308.

Sedbrook, D., "2,4-D: The Most Dangerous Pesticide You've Never Heard Of," March 15, 2016, available at https://www.nrdc.org/stories/24-d-most-dangerous-pesticide-youve-never-heard.

Simon, R. A., "Additive-Induced Urticaria: Experience with Monosodium Glutamate (MSG)," *Journal of Nutrition* 130.4S Supplemental (2000): 1063S-066S. Print.

Strawbridge, H., "Artificial Sweeteners: Sugar-Free, but at What Cost?" January 8, 2018, available at https://www.health.harvard.edu/blog/artificial-sweeteners-sugar-free-but-at-what-cost-201207 165030.

Stromberg, J., "Five Reasons Why You Should Probably Stop Using Antibacterial Soap," January 2014, available at https://www.smithsonianmag.com/science-nature/five-reasons-why-you-should-probably -stop-using-antibacterial-soap-180948078/?no-ist.

Swanson, J. M., and M. Kinsbourne, "Food Dyes Impair Performance of Hyperactive Children on a Laboratory Learning Test," *Science* Vol. 207, Issue 4438 (March 28, 1980): 1485–1487.

Tarazona, et. al., "Glyphosate Toxicity and Carcinogenicity: A Review of the Scientific Basis of the European Union Assessment and Its Differences with IARC," *Archives of Toxicology* 91(8) (2017): 2723–2743.

"2,4-D Herbicide & GMO Crops: Risks to Children from 2,4-D," June 22, 2014, available at https://www .ewg.org/research/24D/risks-to-children-from-24D#.WO4Hi9JKiUl.

"Volatile Organic Compounds' Impact on Indoor Air Quality," United States Environmental Protection Agency, available at https://www.epa.gov/indoor-air-quality-iaq/volatile-organic-compounds-impact -indoor-air-quality.

Weiss, et al., "Behavioral Responses to Artificial Food Colors," *Science* Vol. 207, Issue 4438 (March 28, 1980): 1487–1489.

Yang, C., S. Yaniger, et al., "Most Plastic Products Release Estrogenic Chemicals: A Potential Health Problem That Can Be Solved," *Environmental Health Perspectives* 119(7) (July 2011): 989–996.

Yang, W. H., M. A. Drouin, M. Herbert, Y. Mao, and J. Karsh, "The Monosodium Glutamate Symptom Complex: Assessment in a Double-Blind, Placebo-Controlled, Randomized Study," *The Journal of Allergy and Clinical Immunology* Part 1 99.6 (1997): 757–62. Print.

Zhang, J. S., J. S. Zhang, Q. Chen, and X. Yang, "A Critical Review on Studies of Volatile Organic Compound (VOC) Sorption by Building Materials," *ASHRAE Transactions* 108(1) (2002): 162–174.

Zorrilla, et. al., "The Effects of Triclosan on Puberty and Thyroid Hormones in Male Wistar Rats," *Toxicological Sciences* Volume 107 (1) (January 2009): 56–64.

Chapter 3

Boseley, S., "Sugar, Not Fat, Exposed as Deadly Villain in Obesity Epidemic," *The Guardian,* March 20, 2013, https://www.theguardian.com/society/2013/mar/20/sugar-deadly-obesity-epidemic.

Fallon, S., and M. G. Enig, "The Great Con-ola," July 28, 2002, available at https://www.westonaprice .org/health-topics/know-your-fats/the-great-con-ola/.

Hyman, M., "Why Vegetable Oils Should Not Be Part of Your Diet," *Eco Watch*, February 2, 2016, available at https://www.ecowatch.com/dr-mark-hyman-why-vegetable-oils-should-not-be-part-of -your-diet-1882164589.html.

Mercola, J., "Fructose: This Addictive Commonly Used Food Feeds Cancer Cells, Triggers Weight Gain, and Promotes Premature Aging," April 20, 2010, available at https://articles.mercola.com/sites/ articles/archive/2010/04/20/sugar-dangers.aspx.

Park, A., "When Vegetable Oil Isn't as Healthy as You Think," *Time Magazine,* April 12, 2015, available at http://time.com/4291505/when-vegetable-oil-isnt-as-healthy-as-you-think/.

"The Dangers of Polyunsaturated Vegetable Oils," available at https://www.healingnaturallybybee .com/the-dangers-of-polyunsaturated-vegetable-oils/.

"The Harmful Effects of Sugar on Mind and Body," available at https://rense.com/general45/sguar.htm.

Chapter 10

Amith, H., V. Anil, V. Ankola, and L. Nagesh, "Effect of Oil Pulling on Plaque and Gingivitis," *Journal of Oral Health & Community Dentistry* 1(1) (2007): 12–18.

Anand, T. D., C. Pothiraj, R. M. Gopinath, et al., "Effect of Oil-Pulling on Dental Caries Causing Bacteria [(PDF])," *African Journal of Microbiology Research* 2(3) (March 2008): 63–666.

Asokan, S., J. Rathan, M. S. Muthu, P. V. Rathna, P. Emmadi, Raghuraman, and Chamundeswari, "Effect of Oil Pulling on *Streptococcus mutans* Count in Plaque and Saliva Using Dentocult SM Strip *mutans* Test: A Randomized, Controlled, Triple-Blind Study," *Journal of the Indian Society of Pedodontics & Preventive Dentistry* 26(1) (March 2008): 12-7.

"Gum Disease," Ora Wellness, available at https://www.orawellness.com/prevent-reverse/gum -disease/.

Thaweboon, S., J. Nakaparksin, and B. Thaweboon, "Effect of Oil-Pulling on Oral Microorganisms in Biofilm Models," *Asia Journal of Public Health,* May–August 2011.

Chapter 11

Borax Material Safety Data Sheet, available at https://omsi.edu/sites/all/FTP/files/kids/Borax-msds .pdf.

"Getting to the Bottom of Borax: Is it Safe or Not?," available at https://crunchybetty.com/getting-to -the-bottom-of-borax-is-it-safe-or-not/.

Chapter 12

Cincinelli, A., and T. Martellini, "Indoor Air Quality and Health," *International Journal of Environmental Research and Public Health* 14(11) (November 2017): 1286.

"Public Health, Environmental and Social Determinants of Health," World Health Organization, available at http://www.who.int/phe/health_topics/outdoorair/databases/en/.

Wade, Willard A. III, William A. Cote, and John E. Yocom, "A Study of Indoor Air Quality," *Journal of the Air Pollution Control Association* 25:9 (1975): 933–939.

Chapter 13

Eadicicco, L., "Americans Check Their Phones 8 Billion Times a Day," *Time,* December 15, 2015, available at http://time.com/4147614/smartphone-usage-us-2015/.

Kirkova, D., "Tech Is Taking Over the Dinner Table," *Daily Mail*, September 25, 2014, available at http://www.dailymail.co.uk/femail/article-2769436/Tech-taking-dinner-table-THIRD-kids-distracted-phones-meal-times-social-media-sites-biggest-draw.html.

Maynard, M., "Millennials in 2014: Take My Car, Not My Phone," *Forbes*, January 24, 2014, available at https://www.forbes.com/sites/michelinemaynard/2014/01/24/millenials-in-2014-take-my-car-not-my-phone/.

Siegler, M. G., "Eric Schmidt: Every 2 Days We Create as Much Information as We Did Up to 2003," *TechCrunch*, August 4, 2014, available at https://techcrunch.com/2010/08/04/schmidt-data/.

Chapter 15

Barlow, J., "Children with ADHD Benefit from Time Outdoors Enjoying Nature," *Illinois News Bureau*, August 27, 2004, available at https://news.illinois.edu/view/6367/207524.

"Health and Wellness Benefits of Spending Time in Nature," U.S. Department of Agriculture, Forest Service, available at https://www.fs.fed.us/pnw/about/programs/gsv/pdfs/health_and_wellness.pdf.

Chapter 16

Aamodt, S., and S. Wang, "The Sun Is the Best Optometrist," *New York Times*, June 20, 2011, available at https://www.nytimes.com/2011/06/21/opinion/21wang.html.

Bittner, A. C., R. M. Croffut, M. C. Stranahan, and T. N. Yokelson, "Prescript-Assist Probiotic-Prebiotic Treatment for Irritable Bowel Syndrome: an Open-Label, Partially Controlled, 1-year Extension of a Previously Published Controlled Clinical Trial," *Clinical Therapeutics* 29 (6) (June 2007): 1153–60.

Bittner, A. C., R. M. Croffut, and M. C. Stranahan, "Prescript-Assist Probiotic-Prebiotic Treatment for Irritable Bowel Syndrome: A Methodologically Oriented, 2-Week, Randomized, Placebo-Controlled, Double-Blind Clinical Study," *Clinical Therapeutics* 27(6) (June 2005): 755–61.

Brody, J., "Babies Know: A Little Dirt Is Good for You," *New York Times*, January 6, 2009, available at https://www.nytimes.com/2009/01/27/health/27brod.html.

Callahan, A., "Why Is Breast Milk So Low in Iron? The Science of Mom," October 2011, available at https://scienceofmom.com/2011/10/12/why-is-breast-milk-so-low-in-iron/.

Hallberg, L., and E. Björn-Rasmussen, "Measurement of Iron Absorption from Meals Contaminated with Iron," *The American Journal of Clinical Nutrition* 34(12) (December 1981): 2808–15.

Holbreich, et. al., "Amish Children Living in Northern Indiana Have a Very Low Prevalence of Allergic Sensitization," *The Journal of Allergy and Clinical Immunology* 129 (6) (June 2012): 1671–1673.

"It's in the Dirt! Bacteria in Soil May Make Us Happier, Smarter," Therapeutic Landscapes Network, available at http://www.healinglandscapes.org/blog/2011/01/its-in-the-dirt-bacteria-in-soil-makes-us-happier-smarter/.

Kanter, R., "Trees, Green Space, and Human Well-Being," University of Illinois, July 7, 2005, available at http://lhhl.illinois.edu/media/2005.07_kanter.htm.

Park, B. J., Y. Tsunetsugu, T. Kasetani, T. Kagawa, and Y. Miyazaki, "The Physiological Effects of Shinrin-yoku (Taking in the Forest Atmosphere or Forest Bathing): Evidence from Field Experiments in 24 Forests Across Japan," *Environmental Health and Preventative Medicine* 15(1) (January 2010): 18–26.

Sisson, M., "Forest Bathing," Mark's Daily Apple, July 16, 2010, available at https://www.marksdailyapple.com/forest-bathing/.

Chapter 18

Dvorsky, G., "Why We Need to Sleep In Total Darkness," Gizmodo, January 8, 2014, available at https://io9.gizmodo.com/why-we-need-to-sleep-in-total-darkness-1497075228.

Also by Katie Wells

TAKE THE GUESSWORK OUT OF DINNER

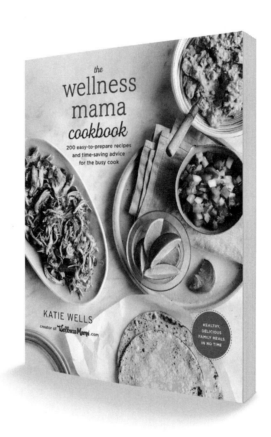

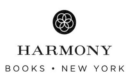

HARMONY

BOOKS · NEW YORK

AVAILABLE EVERYWHERE BOOKS ARE SOLD.